THE HEALTHY SNACKS COLLECTION

By Victoria Love

Edited by Daniel Amos and Sylvie Johnstone

Table of Contents

Cooking Light in 3 Steps

73 Cooking Light 3 Steps or Less Recipes; Fast-n-Light Done Right Meals, Recipes & Cookbook

3 STEP SOUP MEALS
Mushroom and Quinoa Soup

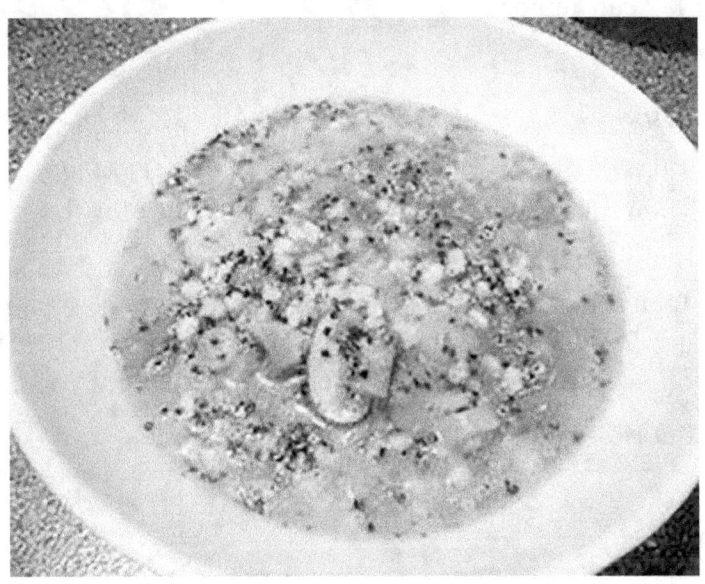

Ingredients

- 7 1/4 cups vegetable broth, low sodium
- 1 cup onion, chopped
- 2 garlic cloves, minced
- 1 medium carrot, peeled and sliced
- 1/2 cup pearl barley
- 2 cups canned tomatoes, low sodium, drained and chopped
- 2 bay leaves
- 1 teaspoon honey

- 1/2 teaspoon ground black pepper
- 1 teaspoon dried basil
- 1 cup mushroom, sliced
- 1/2 cup quinoa

Directions

1. Take a large size pot and heat in this pot, 1/4 cup of broth. Then take garlic, onion and add them. Fry for three min or till onions gets tender.

2. Take the rest of the ingredients and add them, heat to boiling. Lower the temperature, and let it simmer for 50 min or till everything is soften, covered, mix frequently.

3. Get rid of the bay leaves.

Barley Burger Stew for 2

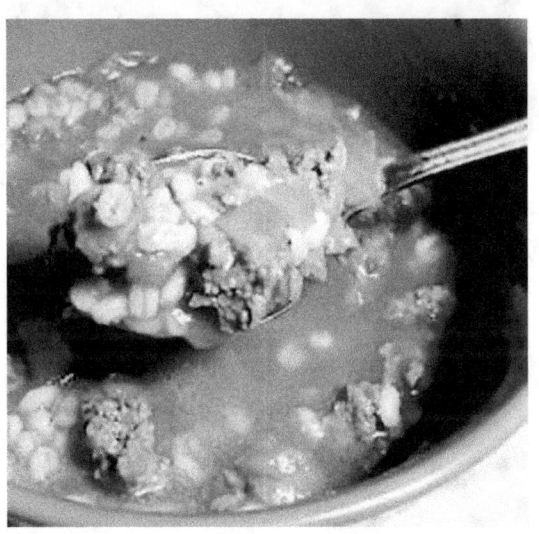

Directions

- 1/2 lb. lean ground beef
- 1/4 cup chopped onion
- 1/4 cup chopped celery
- 2 1/4 cups tomato juice
- 1/2 cup water
- 1/4 cup medium pearl barley
- 1 teaspoon chili powder
- 1/2 teaspoon salt
- 1/2 teaspoon pepper

Directions

1. First of all, take celery, onion and beef AND COOK them in saucepan till pink color disappears, then drain well.

2. Then mix in tomato juice. Then mix in barley. Then mix in chili powder. Then mix in salt. Then mix in pepper. Heat to boiling.

3. Lower the temperature and let it simmer for ONE hour till barley is soften, covered.

Beef Minestrone

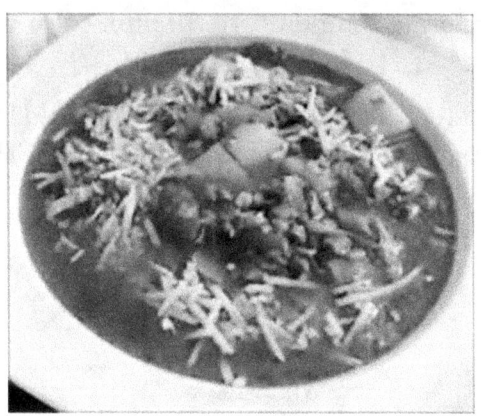

Ingredients

- 1 lb. lean ground beef
- 1 cup onion, chopped
- 6 cups water
- 1 cup potato, peeled chopped
- 1 cup tomato, chopped
- 1 cup cabbage, shredded
- 1 cup carrot, chopped
- 1/2 cup celery, chopped
- 1/4 cup long grain rice, uncooked
- 1/2 teaspoon dried thyme
- 1 bay leaf
- 1/4 teaspoon pepper
- 5 teaspoons parmesan cheese, grated

Directions

1. First of all, take onion, beef and cook them in Dutch oven over moderate temperature till pink color of the meat gets disappear.

2. Take potatoes, bay leaf, and thyme and add them. Then take cabbage, celery, rice and add them as well. Then take water, potatoes and add them too and simmer for SIXTY min.

3. Get rid of the bay leaf. Use half teaspoon of parmesan as sprinkle for every serving.

Green Veggies Soup

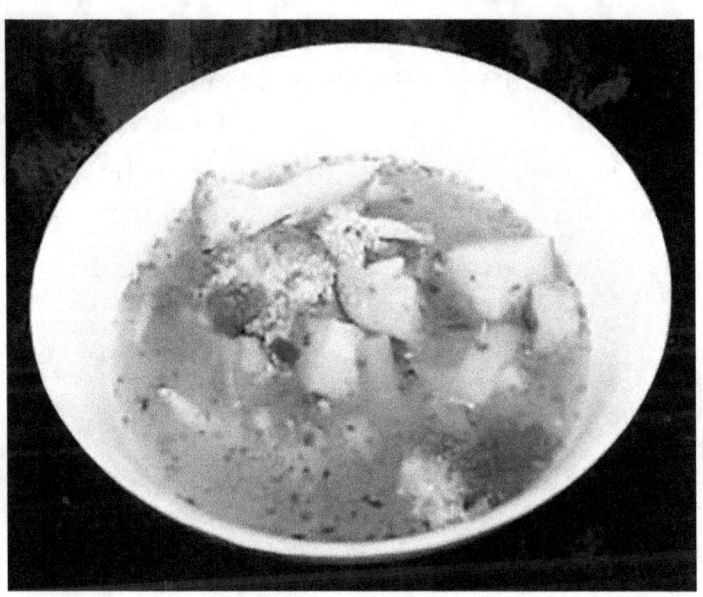

Ingredients

- 1 cup green beans, cut in pieces of 1/2 inch
- 1 tablespoon olive oil
- 2 cups broccoli florets
- 1 cup zucchini, diced
- 3 green onions, finely chopped
- 5 cups chicken stock
- 2 tablespoons pesto sauce
- Pepper

Directions

1. Take green beans and brown them in oil in saucepan for approximately FOUR min at moderate temperature.

2. Take the rest of vegetables and add them and continue cooking for ONE min. Take pesto, chicken stock and add them.

3. Heat to boiling and allow to simmer for three min or till broccoli gets soften. Take pepper and add it.

Cajun Shrimp and Corn Chowder

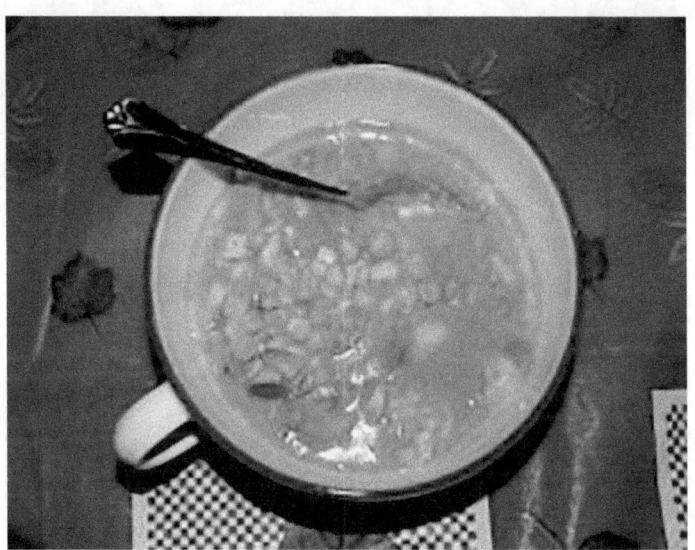

Ingredients

- 1/2 cup butter
- 1 large yellow onion, julienned
- 2 (15 1/4 ounce) cans whole kernel corn
- 2 cups chicken stock
- 2 cups whipping cream
- 1 tablespoon Cajun seasoning
- 6 ounces bay shrimp

Directions

1. Take butter and melt it in medium size saucepan. Take onions and add them fry them till translucent.

2. Take whipping cream along with chicken stock, corn and add them. Let it simmer for THIRTY min. take away from temperature and puree in a blender.

3. Bring it back to pan. Take bay shrimp, Cajun seasoning and add them both, blend well. Allow set for SIXTY min for developing the flavor and then heat again and deliciously serve this recipe.

Leek, Potato, and Tarragon Soup

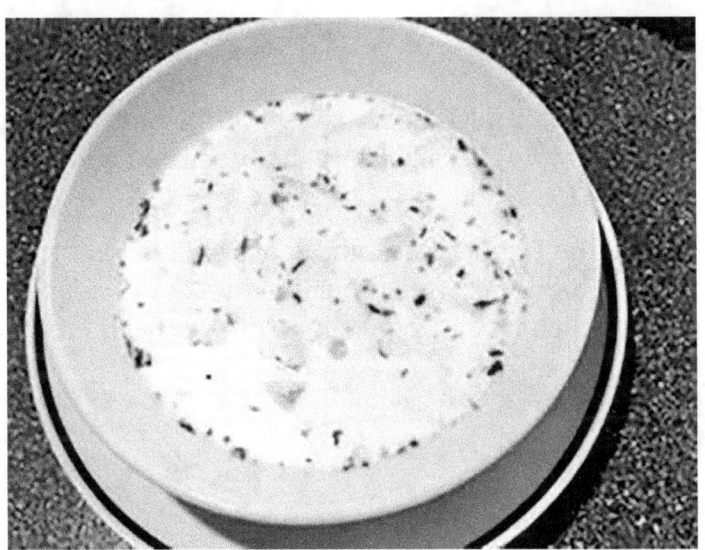

Ingredients

- 3 tablespoons butter
- 2 leeks, sliced (white and pale green parts only)
- 1 small onion, chopped
- 4 garlic cloves, sliced
- 2 tablespoons water
- 1/2 lb. red potatoes, unpeeled, cut into 1/2-inch pieces
- 4 cups low sodium chicken broth or 4 cups vegetable broth
- 2 teaspoons fresh tarragon, chopped
- 1/2 cup whipping cream
- 1/2 cup plain yogurt

Directions

1. First of all, melt butter over moderate temperature in large size heavy pot. Take garlic, onion, two tablespoon water, leeks and add them.

2. Then cook for next ten min or till the color of leeks changes to golden brown. Take broth, potatoes and add them. Heat to boiling.

3. Lower the temperature and let it simmer for ten min or till potatoes get soften. Then mix in tarragon. Then mix in cream. Then mix in yogurt. Use salt, pepper as seasonings.

Potato Cabbage Soup

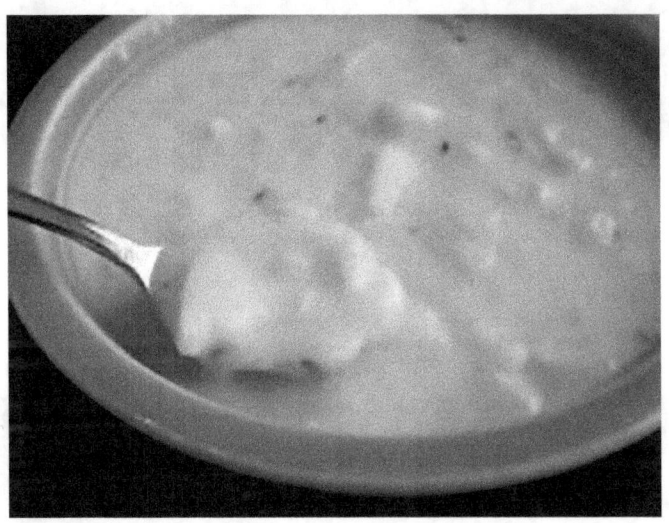

Ingredients

- 1 large onion, chopped
- 2 tablespoons butter
- 10 cups water
- 6 cups chopped cabbage
- 4 cups diced potatoes
- 4 tablespoons chicken bouillon
- 1 tablespoon minced garlic
- 1/2 teaspoon pepper
- 1/2 teaspoon thyme
- 1/8 teaspoon marjoram
- 1/8 teaspoon celery seed

Directions

1. First of all, quick fry onion in butter in large size pot, till soften.

2. Then take the rest of the ingredients and add them all.

3. Let it simmer for TWENTY FIVE min, covered.

White Bean Chili

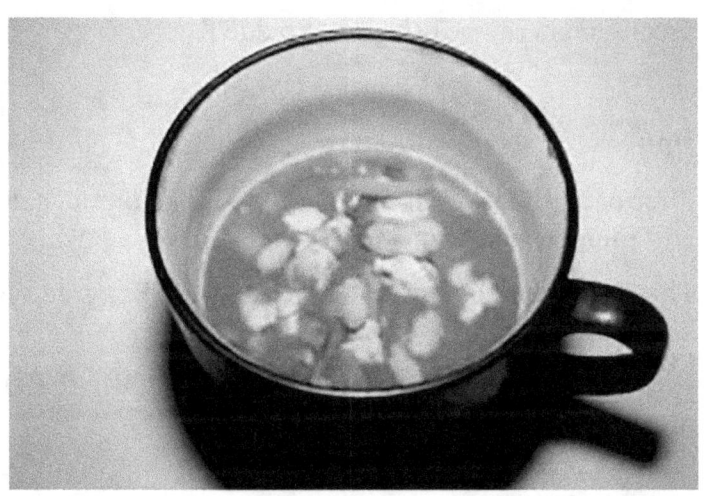

Ingredients

- 2 diced onions
- 2 minced garlic cloves
- 1 tablespoon olive oil
- 4 cups cooked chicken
- 3 (16 ounce) cans great northern beans, drained
- 5 cups chicken broth
- 2 (4 ounce) cans green chilies, chopped and drained
- 2 tablespoons cumin
- 1 1/2 teaspoons chili powder
- 1/4 teaspoon cayenne pepper
- 1/4 teaspoon oregano

- 1/4 teaspoon ground cloves
- 1/8 teaspoon paprika
- 2 cups monterey jack cheese, shredded

Directions

1. First of all, heat oil in the soup pot. Take onion, garlic and add them as well. Quick fry till soften.

2. Then take chicken and the following NINE ingredients and add them as well.

3. Heat to boiling and then let it simmer for THIRTY TO SIXTY min. Use cheese for topping.

Wild Rice and Turkey Stew

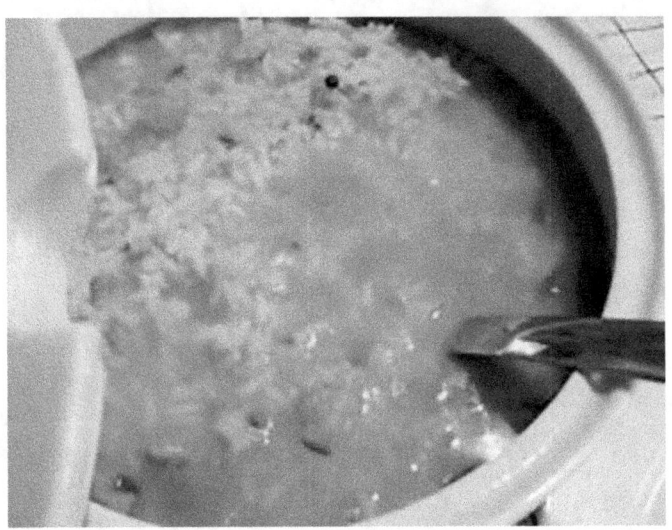

Ingredients

- 1 cup wild rice
- 3 lbs. skinless boneless turkey breasts or 3 lbs. boneless skinless chicken breasts, cubed
- 1 onion, chopped (about 1 cup)
- 1 cup celery heart, chopped
- 4 cups low sodium chicken broth (1 carton)
- 3 tablespoons all-purpose flour
- 3 garlic cloves, minced
- 2 teaspoons dried Italian seasoning
- 1/2 teaspoon pepper, freshly ground
- 2 tablespoons fresh parsley, chopped, to garnish

Directions

1. Take rice, celery, onion, turkey and chicken adding them to slow cooker.

2. Then take one more bowl, whisk together in this bowl, pepper, Italian seasoning, broth, flour, and garlic and then add to the slow cooker.

3. Cook on low temperature for FIVE hours or till turkey/chicken is cooked through. You can serve this recipe with fresh parsley.

Chicken Noodle Soup

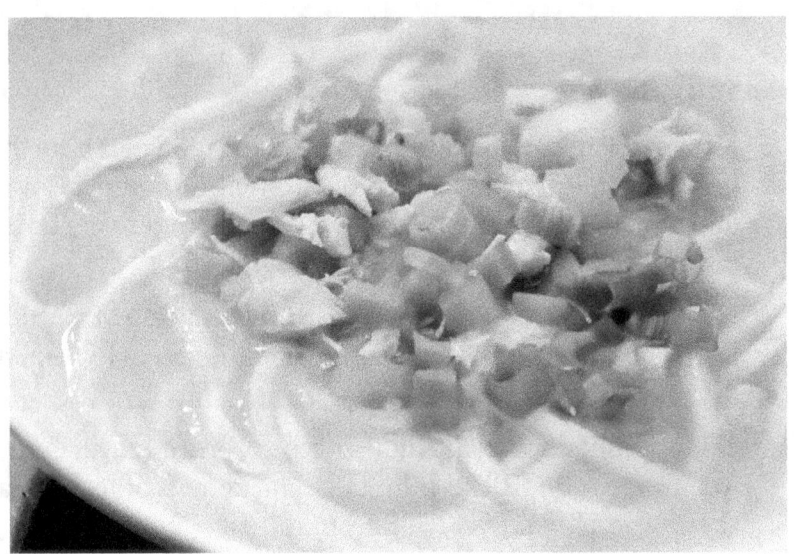

Ingredients

- 1 (3 -4 lb.) broiler-fryer chickens
- 8 -10 cups water
- 1 bay leaf
- 1 tablespoon chopped fresh parsley
- 1 1/4 teaspoons salt
- 1/4 teaspoon pepper
- 1/4 teaspoon dried basil
- 1/8 teaspoon celery seed
- 1/8 teaspoon garlic powder
- 4 medium carrots, chopped

- 1 small onion, chopped
- 1 cup uncooked fine egg noodles

Directions

1. First of all, take the 1st NINE ingredients and combine them together in large size Dutch oven. Heat to boiling. Cover it and lower the temperature and let it simmer for THIRTY min till soften.

2. After this, take out chicken from broth and get rid of the bay leaf. Then right after this, remove skin, bone chicken, and dice meat; and keep aside.

3. Take onion, carrot and add them to broth, cover and let it simmer for THIRTY min. take chicken, noodles and add them. Cook for extra FIFTEEN minutes.

3 Step Main Dish Meals
Best Grilled Pork Chops

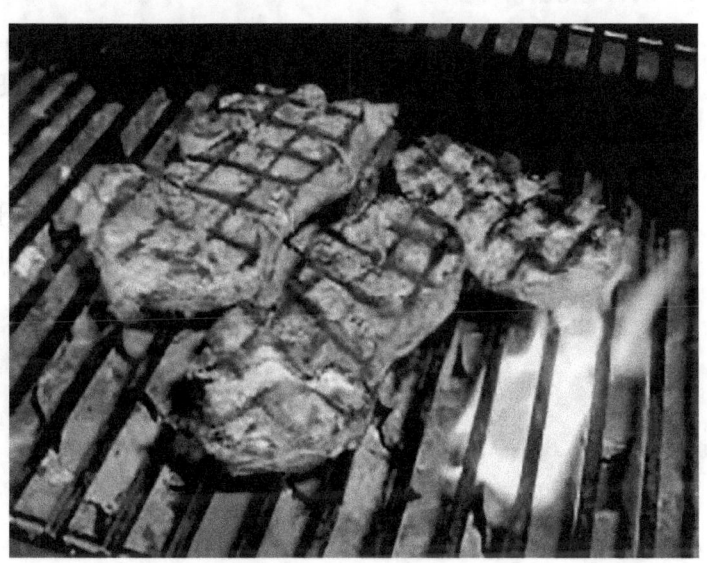

Ingredients

- 1/2 cup water
- 1/3 cup light soy sauce
- 1/4 cup vegetable oil
- 3 tablespoons lemon pepper seasoning
- 2 garlic cloves, minced
- 6 pork loin chops, fat removed

Directions

1. First of all, take all of the marinade ingredients and blend them well in deep bowl and let it marinate for a minimum of TWO hours.

2. Take out from marinade and cook over moderately high temperature on grill that has been greased for FIFTEEN min or till ready and done. The cooking time for the other side is ONE TO TWO min.

3. After this, rotate FORTY FIVE degrees for uniform and equal cooking. Flip over once meat is cooked half way through.

Best Beef Stroganoff

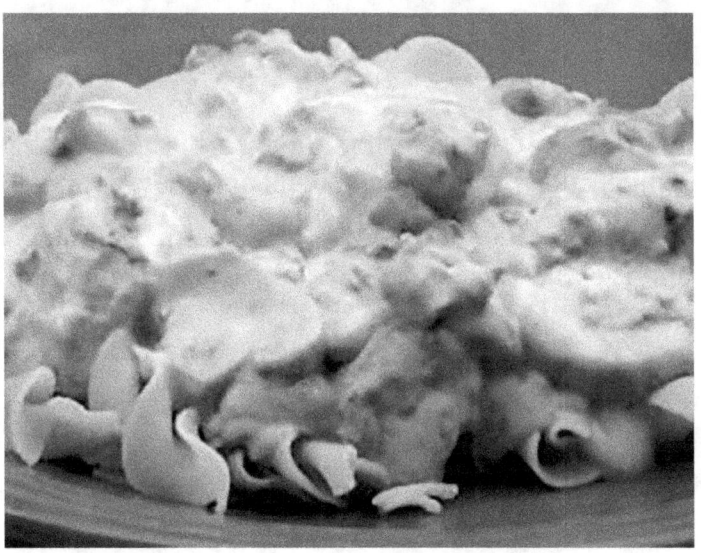

Ingredients

- 1/2 cup minced onion
- 1 cup sour cream
- 1 garlic clove, minced
- 1/4 cup butter
- 1 lb. ground beef
- 2 tablespoons flour
- 1 teaspoon salt
- 1/4 teaspoon pepper
- Canned mushroom stems and pieces, 2-3 cans, drained
- 1 (10 3/4 ounce) cans cream of mushroom soup (I always use

the top name brand)
- 1 (12 ounce) bags egg noodles, cooked

Directions

1. Take garlic, onion and fry them in butter over moderate temperature. Mix in ground beef and brown it well.

2. Then mix in flour. Then mix salt, then mix in mushrooms and then mix in pepper. Cook for five min and then mix in soup.

3. Let it simmer for ten min, uncovered. Mix in sour cream till heated well. You can serve this recipe over noodles.

Chili Con Carne with Beans

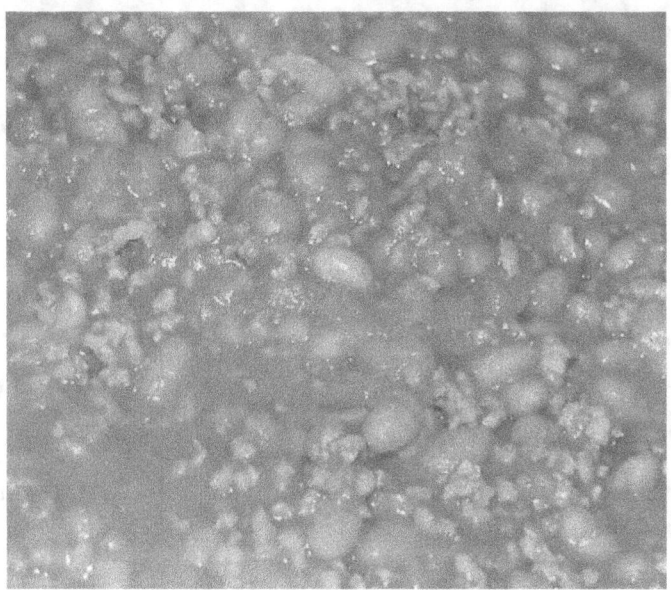

Ingredients

- 2 lbs. ground beef
- 1 large onion, chopped
- 2 garlic cloves, minced
- 1 (15 ounce) cans tomato sauce
- 1 (6 ounce) cans tomato paste
- 1 (15 ounce) cans tomatoes
- 1 (15 ounce) cans diced tomatoes with green chilies
- 1 (12 ounce) bottles dark beer
- 1 teaspoon ground cumin

- 1 teaspoon paprika
- 2 teaspoons chili powder
- 1 teaspoon oregano
- 1 teaspoon salt
- 1/2 teaspoon pepper
- 1 teaspoon Worcestershire sauce
- 1 (28 ounce) cans chili beans

Directions

1. First of all, take garlic, onions, and meat and fry them till ready and done.
2. Take the rest of ingredients and add them. Let it simmer for two hours.

Greek-Style Turkey Burgers

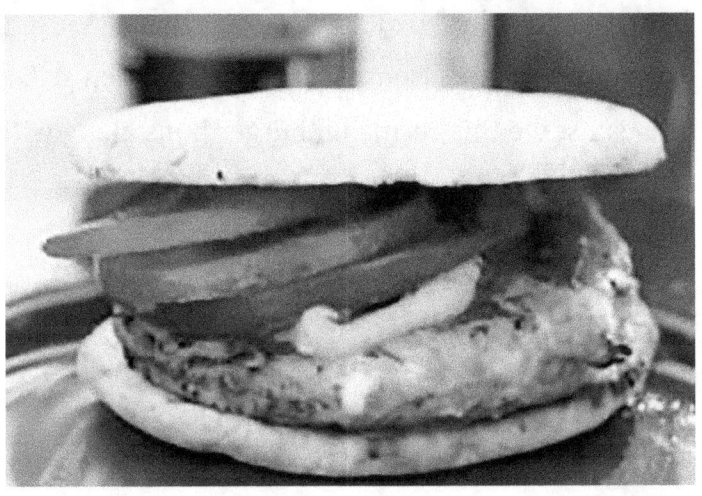

Ingredients

- 1 lb. ground turkey
- 1 cup crumbled feta cheese
- 1/2 cup olive, chopped (Usually I use chopped salad olives)
- 1 teaspoon dried oregano
- 1 teaspoon Italian seasoning
- 1 teaspoon dried parsley
- 1 teaspoon dried basil (optional)
- 1 teaspoon onion powder
- 1/2 teaspoon garlic powder
- Ground black pepper, to taste

Directions

1. First, take a large size bowl, and combine all of the above Ingredients in this bowl.

2. Make FOUR patties from the mixture and then grill them.

3. You can serve this recipe on burger buns along with mayo and tomatoes.

Dirty Shrimp in Butter-Beer Sauce

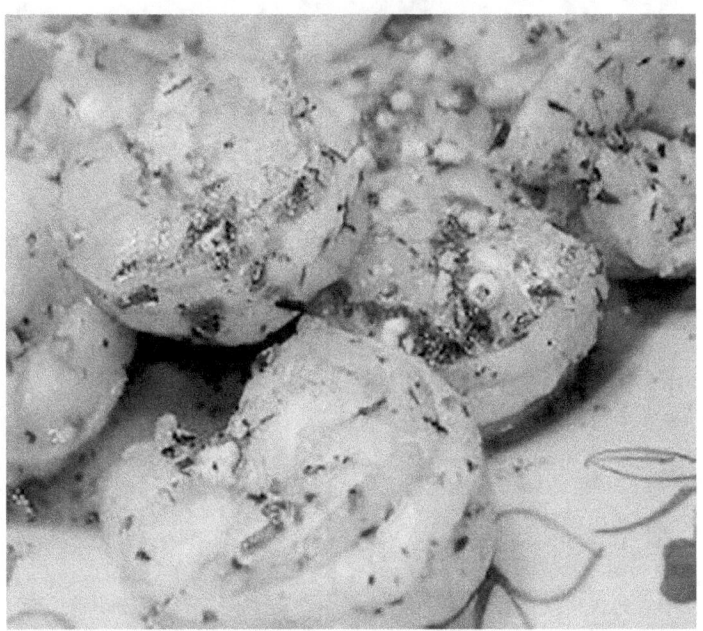

Ingredients

- 2 lbs. shrimp, shelled and deveined
- 4 tablespoons butter
- 2 teaspoons garlic, minced
- 1 teaspoon dried oregano
- 1 teaspoon dried basil
- 1 teaspoon dried thyme
- 1 teaspoon cayenne pepper

- 1/2 teaspoon crushed red pepper flakes
- 1/2 teaspoon salt, to taste
- 1/2 teaspoon black pepper, to taste
- 1/2 cup beer

Directions

1. Take herbs, garlic and fry them in butter till garlic is lightly brown in color.

2. Take shrimp and add it, mix continuously, till shrimp color changes to pink and is ready and done.

3. After this, pour in beer, then let it simmer for ONE min or two. Serve deliciously.

Cheddar Bar-B-Q Chicken Breasts!!!

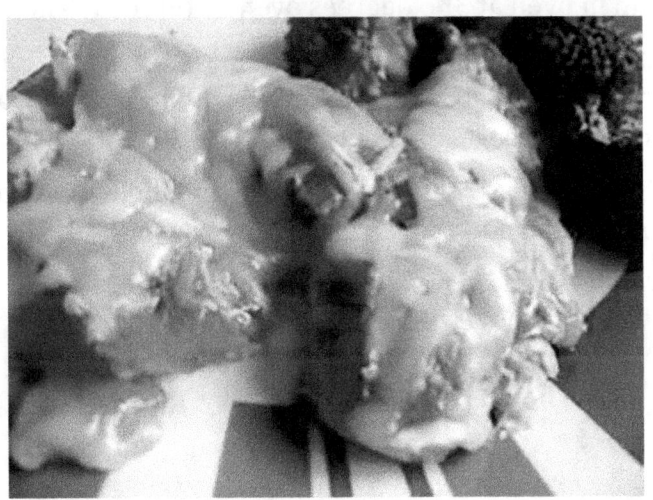

Ingredients

- 4 boneless skinless chicken breasts
- 8 slices cooked bacon
- 1 cup shredded cheddar cheese
- 1/4 cup green onion
- 1 cup barbecue sauce

Directions

1. Take the chicken breasts and cover them with BBQ sauce, then bake them for approximately FIFTEEN TO THIRTY min in oven at 35o degrees oven or till ready and done.

2. After this, pour on additional and extra sauce, take bacon strips and add them for covering the breasts, then again use cheddar cheese for covering.

3. Bring back to oven till cheese gets melted. Take sliced green onions and add them. Your recipe is ready.

Outback Steakhouse® -Style Steak

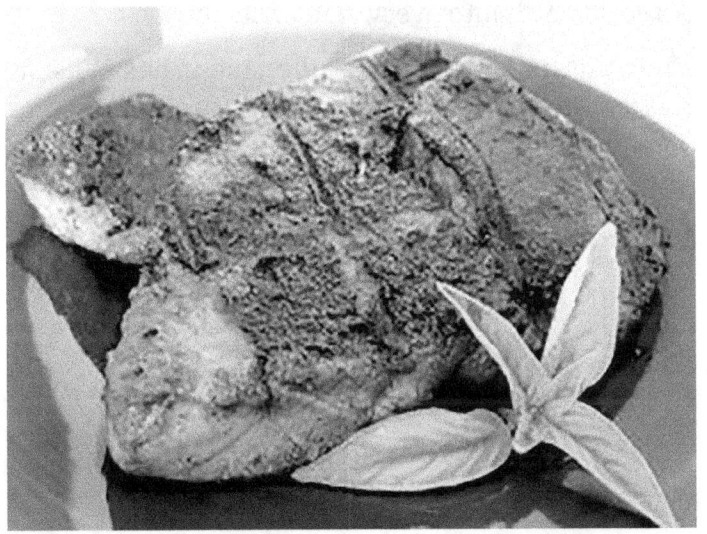

Ingredients

- 4 pieces top sirloin steaks or 4 pieces rib eye steaks
- Seasoning
- 4-6 teaspoons salt (depending on taste)
- 4 teaspoons paprika
- 2 teaspoons ground black pepper
- 1 teaspoon onion powder
- 1 teaspoon garlic powder
- 1 teaspoon cayenne pepper
- 1/2 teaspoon coriander
- 1/2 teaspoon turmeric

Directions

1. Take the seasoning ingredients and blend them together. After this, rub into every side of steak.

2. After this, take large size skillet and grill steaks on it over moderately high temperature, then press down on steak.

Detweiler Sloppy Joe Mix

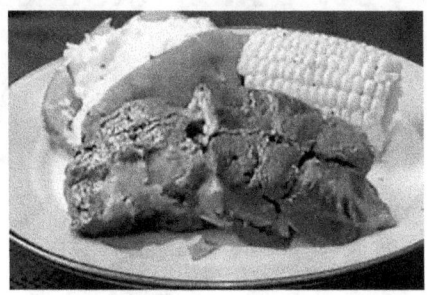

Ingredients

- 1 lb. ground beef
- Onion, chopped (to taste)
- Green pepper, chopped (to taste)
- 1 cup catsup
- 2 tablespoons brown sugar
- 1 tablespoon mustard
- 1/2 cup water

Directions

1. Take green pepper, onion, and hamburger and BROWN THEM together.
2. Then take the rest of ingredients and add them and let it simmer for FIFTEEN min.

Easiest Tastiest Barbecue Country Style Ribs (Slow Cooker)

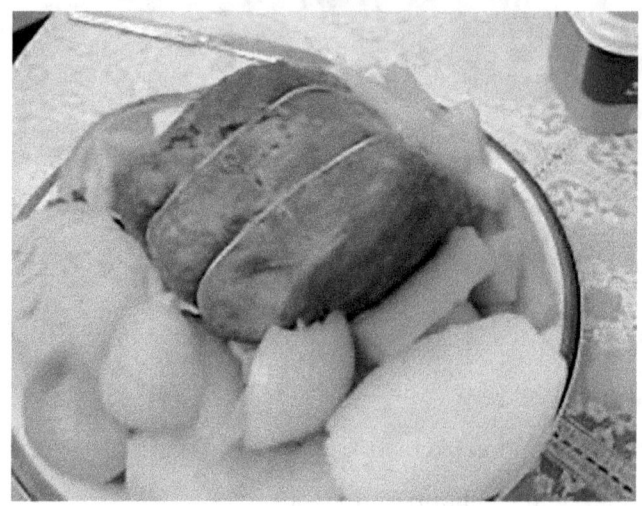

Ingredients

- 4 -5 lbs. country-style pork ribs
- 1 (18 ounce) bottles of your favorite barbecue sauce (I used brown sugar flavor)
- 1 onion, chopped
- Salt and pepper, to taste

Directions

1. Take all of the components/Ingredients and put them all in crockpot.
2. Then cook on low temperature for SIX TO EIGHT hours.
3. After this, you will see meat begins to fall off the ones.

Crock Pot Corned Beef and Cabbage

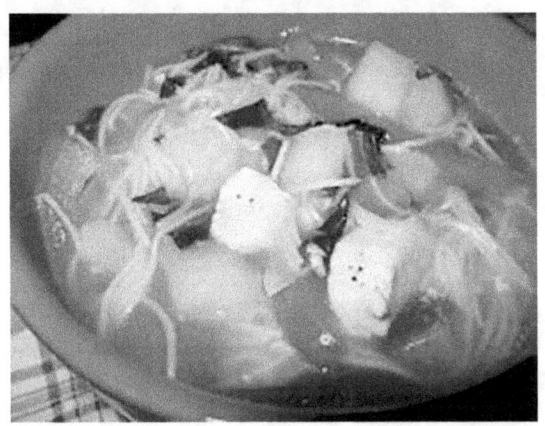

Ingredients

- 4 1/2 lbs. corned beef brisket
- 2 medium onions, quartered
- 1 head cabbage, cut in small wedges
- 1/2 teaspoon pepper
- 3 tablespoons vinegar
- 3 tablespoons sugar
- 2 cups water

Directions

1. Take all of the ingredients and combine them together in crockpot along with cabbage over the top.

2. After this, if required, chop the meat to fit and adjust.

3. Then cook on high temperature for SIX TO SEVEN hours, covered.

3 STEP PASTA MEALS
Tomato Soup & Shells

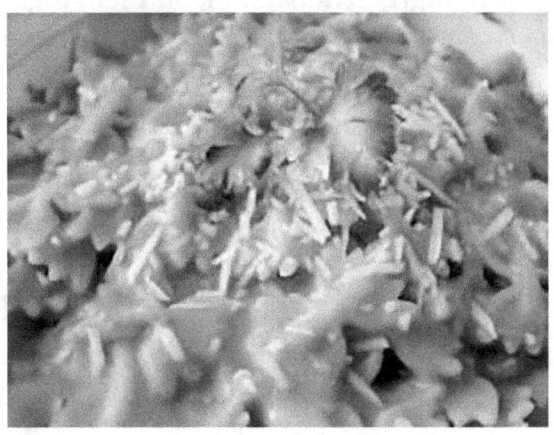

Ingredients

- 7 -8 ounces mini pasta shells, uncooked
- 1 (10 1/2 ounce) cans condensed tomato soup, undiluted
- 5 ounces whipping cream
- 1 -2 ounce Velveeta cheese, cubed
- 1 teaspoon butter
- 1/8-1/4 teaspoon garlic powder
- 1/8-1/4 teaspoon onion powder
- Salt & pepper, to taste

Directions

1. Take shells and place them on boil. Take out from heat when ready and done.

2. Take rest of ingredients and blend them together in small size sauce pan. Let it simmer over low temperature.

3. Then drain the shells well, then take soup and add to shells, mix well.

Pasta Pockets

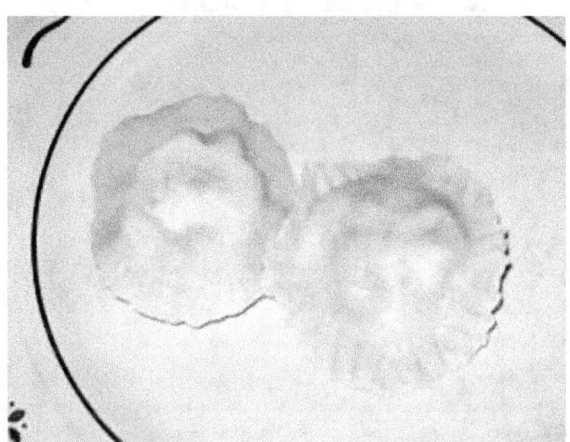

Ingredients

- 1 1/2 cups semolina or 1 1/2 cups bread flour or 1 1/2 cups unbleached all-purpose flour

- 3 eggs

- 1/2 teaspoon salt

- 1 tablespoon olive oil

Directions

1. Take every ingredient above and place them in food processor and pulse well till it pulls away from the container sides. Make a ball from the dough.

2. Knead FIVE TO TEN time on surface that has been coated with flour.

3. Allow to rest for thirty min, use damp towel for covering.

Penne with Chicken & Broccoli Casserole

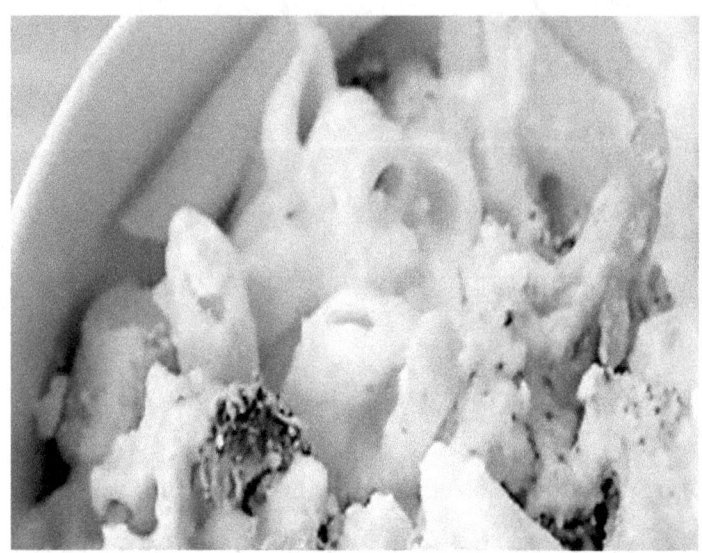

Ingredients

- 1 (16 ounce) boxes penne pasta, cooked (I use less sometimes)
- 2 (16 ounce) jars alfredo sauce, warmed
- 4 cups cheese, shredded & divided in half (4-cheese Mexican blend is good)
- 1 bunch broccoli, cooked (I use a large one)
- 3 -4 boneless skinless chicken breasts, seasoned, cooked, & cut into bite-sized pieces

Directions

1. Take a pan, spray it well. Take a bowl, mix in this bowl, pasta, chicken, broccoli, Alfredo sauce & one bag of the cheese till well mixed.

2. Then right after this, dump into baking pan. Use the rest of bag of cheese and sprinkle all over the top.

3. Then bake for ten min at 35o degrees Fahrenheit or till cheese gets melted.

15 Minute Pasta Combo

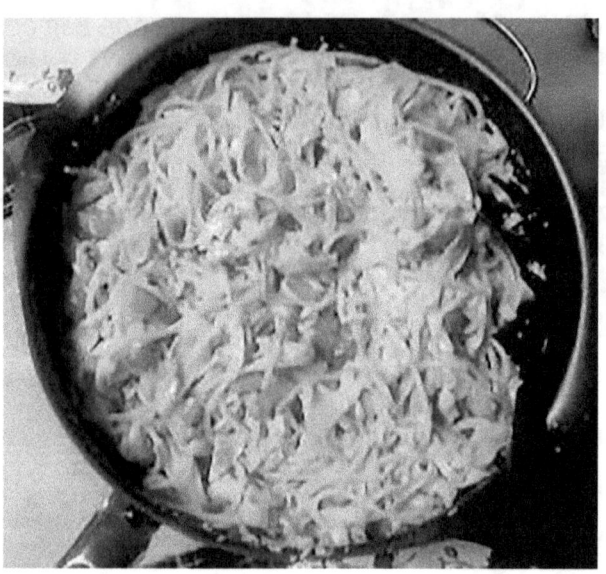

Ingredients

- 8 ounces uncooked spaghetti, broken in half
- 1/2 cup Italian salad dressing
- 2 large fresh tomatoes, seeded and chopped
- 2 cups smoked turkey breast, cubed
- 1 cup grated parmesan cheese

Directions

1. Take spaghetti and cook it till soften. Drain well.

2. Then take the same pan, heat Italian salad dressing in this pan over moderate temperature. Take cooked pasta and add it.

3. Toss well. Add tomatoes. Add turkey. Add parmesan cheese. Toss slightly and lightly.

Spicy Kielbasa Pasta!

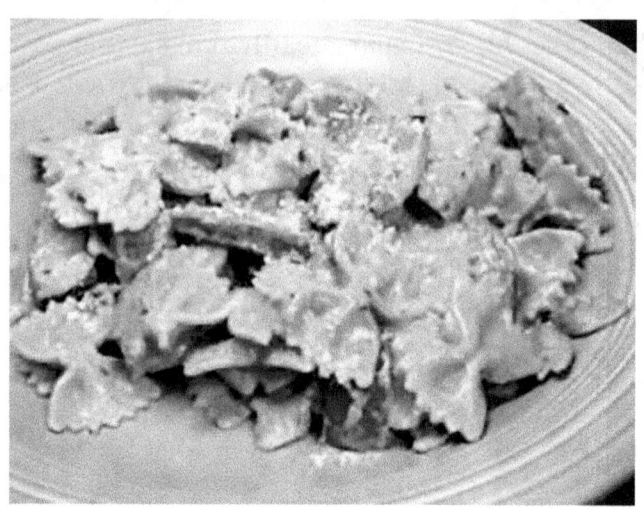

Ingredients

- 2 tablespoons butter
- 2 tablespoons olive oil
- 2 lbs. kielbasa (cut into bite sized pieces)
- 1 (1 lb.) box bow tie pasta (or whatever floats your boat)
- 1 (16 ounce) jars Prego pasta sauce
- 1 (1 ounce) packet crushed red pepper flakes
- 1 red bell pepper (cut into bite sized pieces)
- 1 cup sour cream
- Parmesan cheese, for topping

Directions

1. Take pasta and prepare it as instructed on the package. Drain well. Take butter, olive oil and heat them. Then add kielbasa.

2. Then add crushed pepper. Then add red bell pepper, quick fry till kielbasa change its color to brown.

3. Take the pasta pot, add to this pot, drained pasta along with sour cream , pasta sauce and kielbasa mixture till heated through.

Baked Alpine Noodles and Cheese

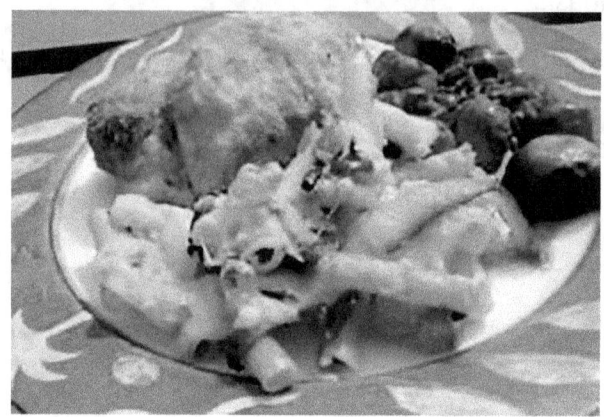

Ingredients

- 1 (1 lb.) package egg noodles
- 1 tablespoon vegetable oil
- 1 tablespoon butter
- 2 ounces mild pancetta or 2 ounces bacon, diced
- 3/4 teaspoon caraway seeds or 3/4 teaspoon cumin seed
- 4 cups onions, thinly sliced
- 1 pinch salt
- 2 eggs
- 3/4 cup milk
- 1 pinch pepper
- 1 pinch nutmeg
- 2 cups shredded ementhal cheese or 2 cups raclette cheese

Directions

1. Take a large size pot and put boiling salted water in this water, cook noodles in this pot as instructed on the package till soften.

2. Drain well and let it chill under water and then drain.

3. Take a frying, and heat oil as well as butter in this frying pan over moderately high temperature. Add pancetta. Then add caraway seeds. Quick fry. Add onions and cook, mix frequently, till become golden brown in color, approximately twelve min. take it away from heat.

4. Take a large size bowl, whisk together in this bowl, eggs, milk, and pepper and nutmeg; and then mix in noodles. Then mix in onion mixture. Then mix in half of the cheese. Then put in buttered baking dish. Use the rest of cheese as sprinkle. Bake for thirty min, at 375 degrees Fahrenheit, uncovered, till it gets lightly brown in color.

Mizithra Browned Butter Pasta

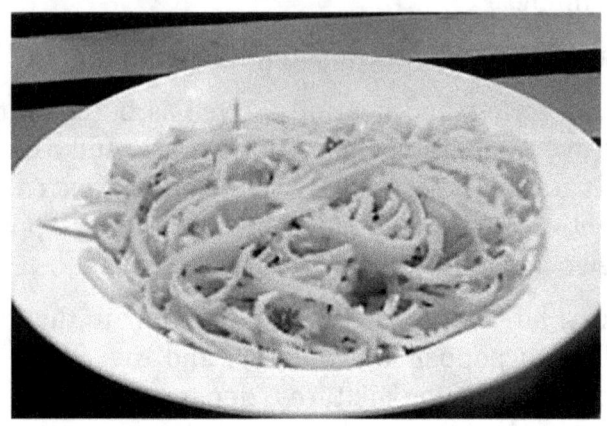

Ingredients

- 1 lb. pasta
- 1/2-1 cup butter or 1/2-1 cup olive oil
- 3 garlic cloves, minced
- 1/2 cup mizithra cheese, grated
- 1/2 cup parmesan cheese, freshly grated
- 1/4 cup chopped fresh parsley
- 1 teaspoon chopped fresh Greek oregano

Directions

1. Take pasta and prepare in large size pot of salted as well as boiling water till ready and done, drain well.

2. Then after this, take butter and melt it over moderate temperature till golden in color. Quick fry garlic. Toss pasta with mixture of garlic and butter.

3. Use cheese and herbs as sprinkles, according to your own choice and taste. Take some of the fresh cracked black pepper use it as sprinkle.

Shrimp and Tomato Pasta

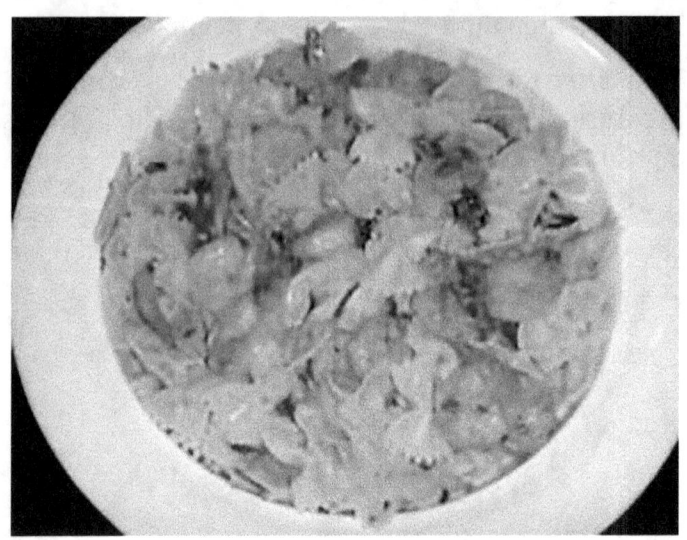

Ingredients

- 1 lb. small shrimp, peeled and deveined
- 4 garlic cloves
- 1/4 cup olive oil
- 1 teaspoon dried basil
- 1/4 teaspoon crushed red pepper flakes
- Salt and pepper
- 3 tablespoons fresh parsley, chopped
- 1 (14 ounce) cans diced tomatoes, undrained
- 1 lb. linguine
- Fresh grated parmesan cheese

Directions

1. Take a large size saucepan, mix in this bowl, basil, crushed red pepper flakes, salt, pepper, parsley, shrimp, garlic, olive oil, and tomatoes in this pan.

2. Let it simmer for ten to fifteen min or till shrimp changes its color to pink. Then take pasta and cook it in another pan, it takes ten to twelve min.

3. Drain the pasta well. And then place them in plates. Use sauce for topping. Use fresh parmesan cheese as sprinkle.

Garlic Parmesan Pasta

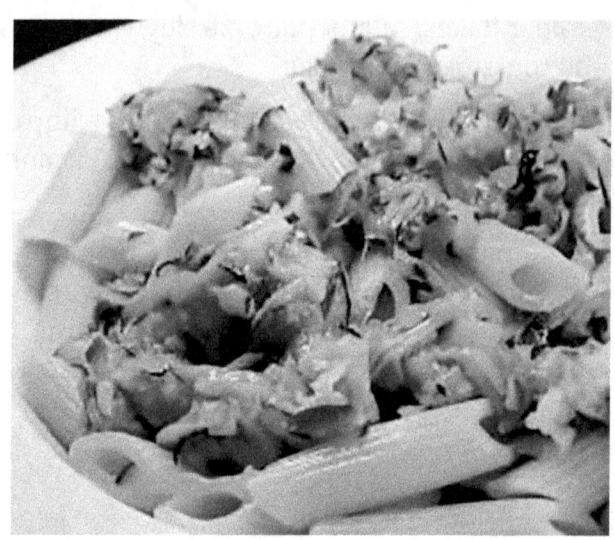

Ingredients

- 1/2 cup margarine
- 2 teaspoons dried basil
- 2 teaspoons lemon juice
- 1 1/4 teaspoons garlic powder
- 3/4 teaspoon seasoning salt
- 8 ounces fettuccine, cooked and drained
- 1 1/2 cups broccoli florets, steamed crisp-tender
- 3 tablespoons walnuts, chopped
- 1/4-1/2 cup parmesan cheese

Directions

1. Take a large size frying pan, melt margarine in this frying pan. Add basil. Then add garlic powder, then add lemon juice. Blend well.

2. Take walnuts along with broccoli, fettuccine and add them. Blend well. Take cheese and add it as well. Toss well.

Spicy Sonora Chicken & Pasta

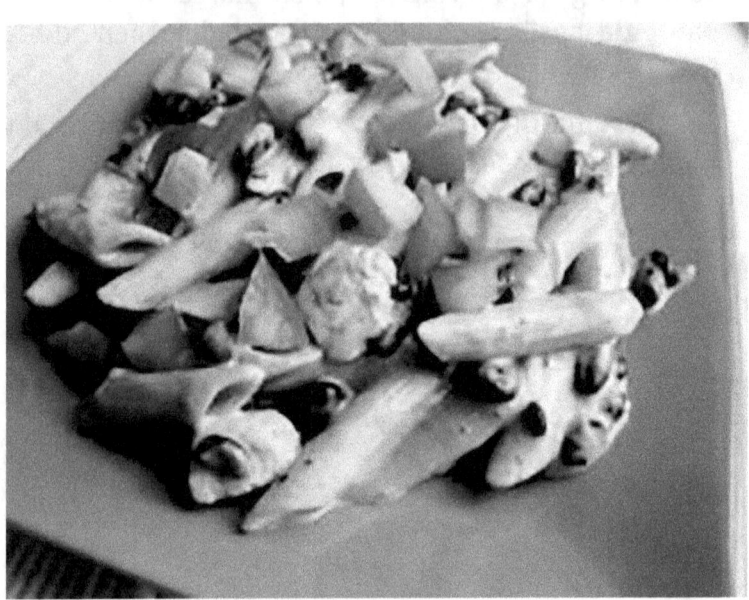

Ingredients

- 1 lb. penne pasta
- 1/2 lb. cooked boneless skinless chicken breast, diced
- 1 (16 ounce) jars white cheese dip (medium or spicy queso dip)
- 1 (15 ounce) cans black beans, drained
- 1 (8 ounce) cans tomato sauce (basil garlic oregano flavor is the best to use)
- 1 tomato, seeded & diced

Directions

1. Take noodles and boil them till soften. Then drain well and place them in large size bowl. Then put cooked chicken in the bowl as well.

2. Take queso dip and heat it along with black beans, tomato sauce in a saucepan. Then take this and pour it over noodles.

3. Use diced tomatoes for topping.

3 STEP BREAKFAST MEALS
Banana Milk

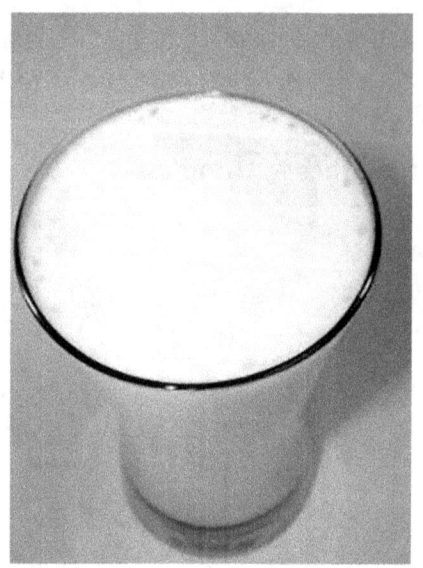

Ingredients

- 1 banana
- 1 cup water or 1 cup milk
- 1/2 teaspoon vanilla

Directions

1. Take all of the ingredients and mix them in a blender till smooth enough.

2. Then take it and pour in glass. Or you can pour over your favorite cereal.

Quick 'n Easy Strawberry and Banana Smoothie

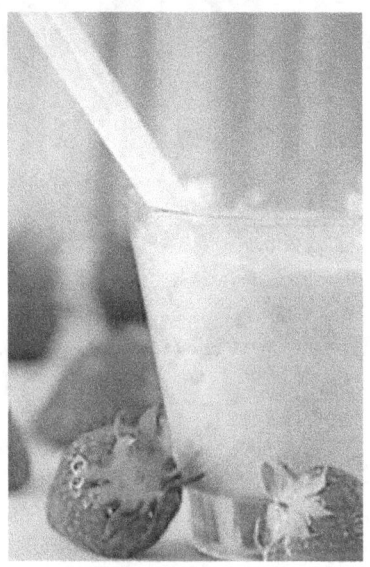

Ingredients

- 250 g strawberries, hulled
- 1 medium banana, peeled and roughly chopped
- 300 ml 1% low-fat milk
- 150 ml natural yoghurt
- 15 ml spoon clear honey

Directions

1. Take all of the above ingredients and put them in a food processor and mix them till smooth enough.

2. When done pour into glasses.

Buttermilk Bran Muffins

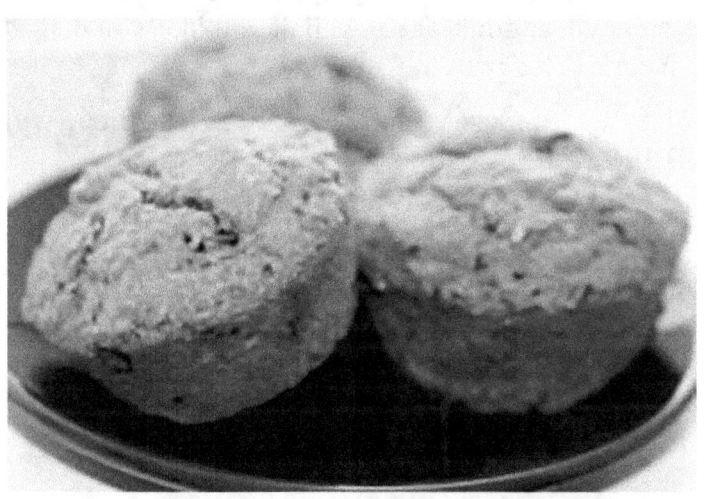

Ingredients

- 2 cups wheat bran (NOT bran cereal)
- 1 cup sugar
- 2 1/2 cups flour
- 2 1/2 teaspoons baking soda
- 1 teaspoon salt
- 1/2 cup oil
- 2 cups buttermilk
- 2 eggs, beaten
- 2 tablespoons molasses

Directions

1. Take the 1st FIVE ingredients and combine them in large size bowl, and mix them well. If you like, you can add your favorite dried fruit in it.

2. Then take greased muffin cups and fill them with TWO THIRD with the batter.

3. Finally, bake them for EIGHTEEN Min at THREE HUNDRED 50 (350) degrees Fahrenheit or till when toothpick comes out neat and clean when inserted in the middle.

Chocolate-Peanut Butter| Smoothie

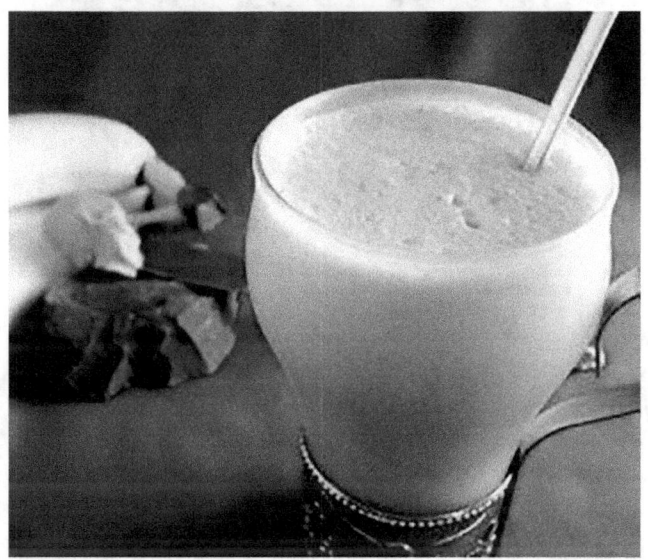

Ingredients

- 1 small ripe banana
- 1 1/2 cups milk
- 1/4 cup smooth peanut butter
- 1/2 teaspoon vanilla extract
- 2 tablespoons chocolate syrup

Directions

1. Take all of the ingredients above and blend them in a food processor till smooth.

Applesauce-Cranberry Oatmeal

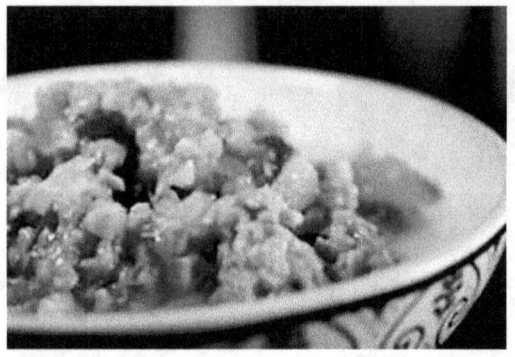

Ingredients

- 3 tablespoons oatmeal, uncooked
- 1 tablespoon dried cranberries
- 1/2 cup unsweetened applesauce
- 1/2 cup water
- 1/8 teaspoon ground cinnamon

Directions

1. Take all of the ingredients and blend them well.
2. Then keep in microwave for TWO min.

Greek Yoghurt and Fruit Salad

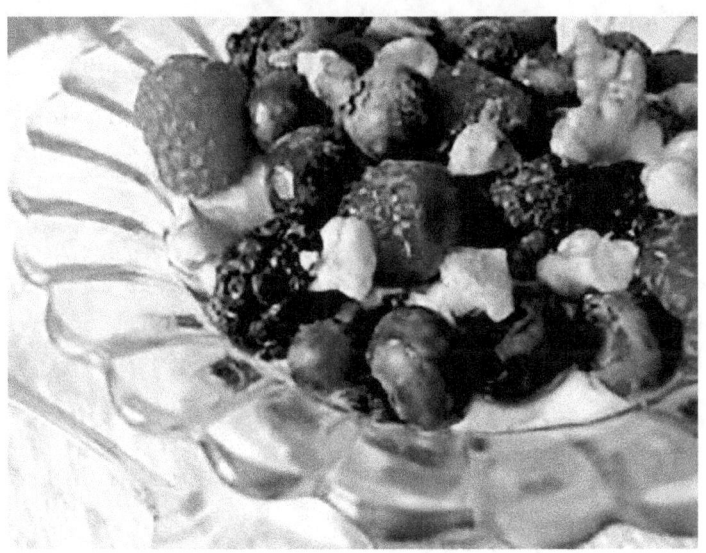

Ingredients

- 200 g Greek yogurt, 8 oz.
- Fresh fruit salad, of your choice
- 2 tablespoons honey
- 4 tablespoons toasted walnut pieces
- Cinnamon

Directions

1. First of all, take a sundae glass and layer in it, some fruit salad and use half of the yogurt as topping for each serving.

2. Then take additional fruit and layer over the top. Use one tablespoon of honey and drizzle over every serving.

3. Use two tablespoons of walnut slices and cinnamon as sprinkles.

Huevos a La Mexicana

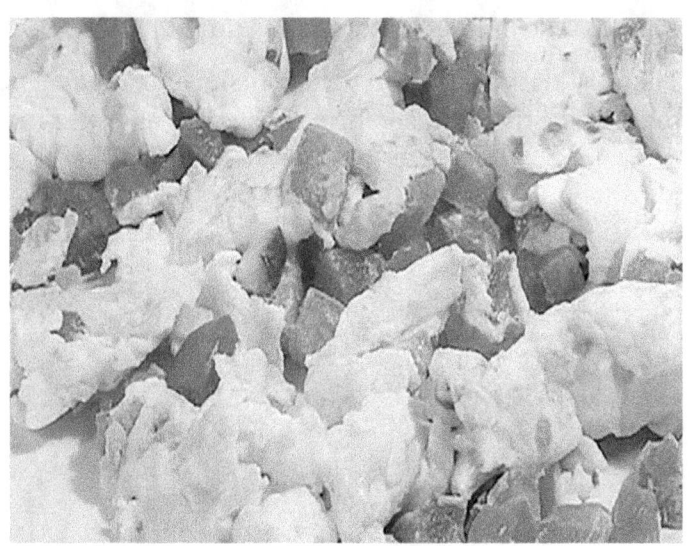

Ingredients

- 4 eggs
- 1 medium sized tomato, washed and diced
- 1/4 onion, finely chopped
- 1 -2 serrano pepper, chopped
- 1 tablespoon butter
- 1 tablespoon oil
- Salt

Directions

1. First of all, take a deep frying and melt in this pan, butter and oil, take peppers, onion and add them.

2. Then fry them till onion gets translucent. Take eggs, tomato and add them, mix continuously. Till eggs are ready and done.

3. Use salt according to your taste as seasoning.

Blueberry Blast Breakfast Smoothie

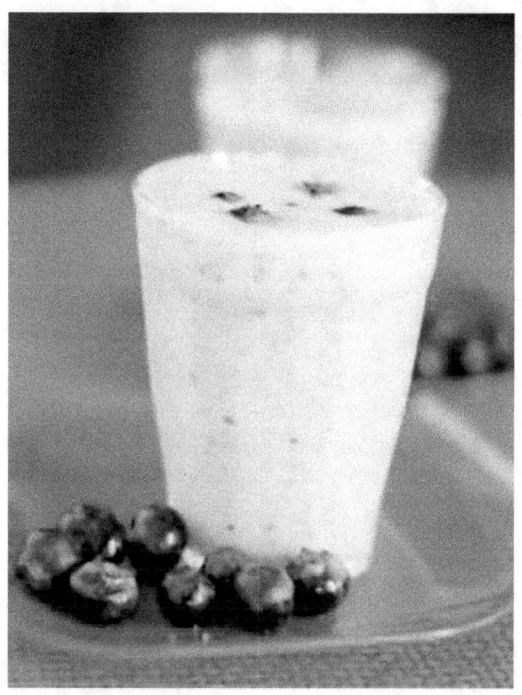

Ingredients

- 2/3 cup frozen blueberries or 2/3 cup fresh blueberries
- 1/2 cup organic vanilla yogurt (can use fat free)
- 1 banana
- 1/2 cup cold fruit juice, your choice
- 1 tablespoon wheat germ

Directions

1. First of all, take all of the above ingredients and put them in a blender and mix them till

Bailey's Irish Cream Fruit Dip

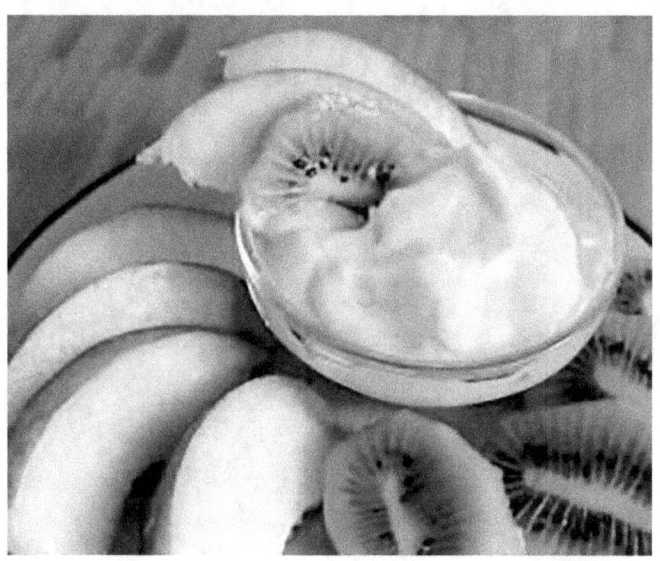

Ingredients

- 1 (6 ounce) packages instant vanilla pudding
- 1 cup milk
- 1/2 cup Bailey's Irish Cream
- 1 (8 ounce) containers Cool Whip

Directions

1. Take all of the components and ingredients and WHIP THEM TOGETHER.
2. You can either serve this recipe right away or chill it.

Breakfast Mock Cinnabon (Low Carb)

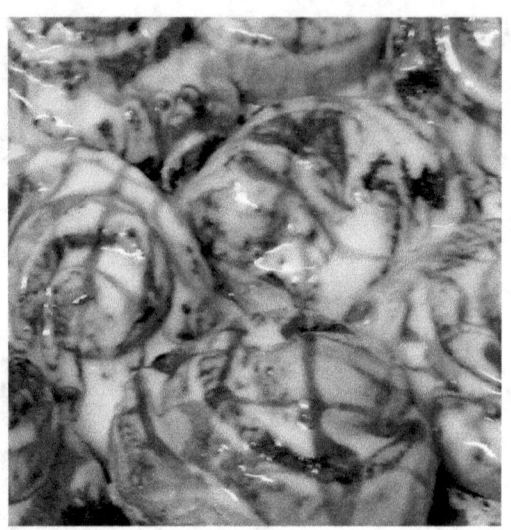

Ingredients

- 1/2 cup 1% fat cottage cheese
- 1 (1 g) packet sugar substitute
- 7 pecan halves, toasted if you prefer
- Ground cinnamon

Directions

1. First of all, take sugar substitute, cottage cheese and combine them together well.
2. You can use cinnamon as sprinkle. And use pecan halves as toppings.

3 STEP SIDE DISH MEALS
Mom's Famous Crock Pot Cream Corn

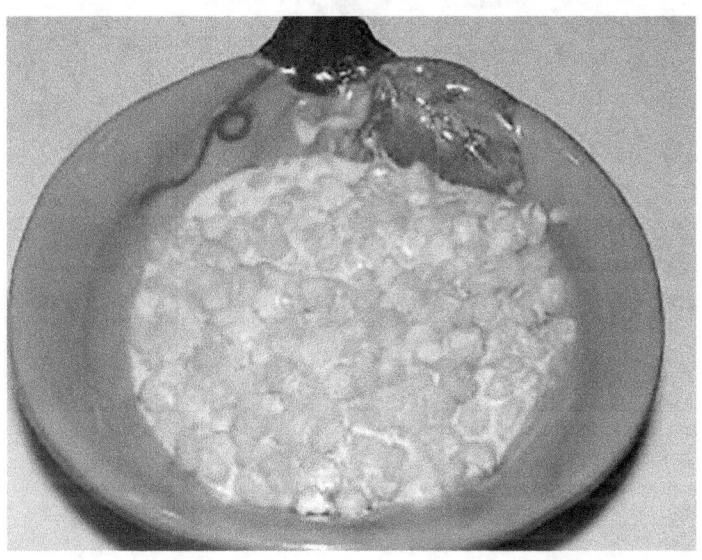

Ingredients

- 20 ounces frozen corn
- 1/2 cup oleo
- 1 (8 ounce) packages cream cheese
- 1 1/2 tablespoons sugar

Directions

1. First of all, cook on low temperature for approximately four hours, mix frequently till all of the components are mixed.

Cherry Tomato Salad

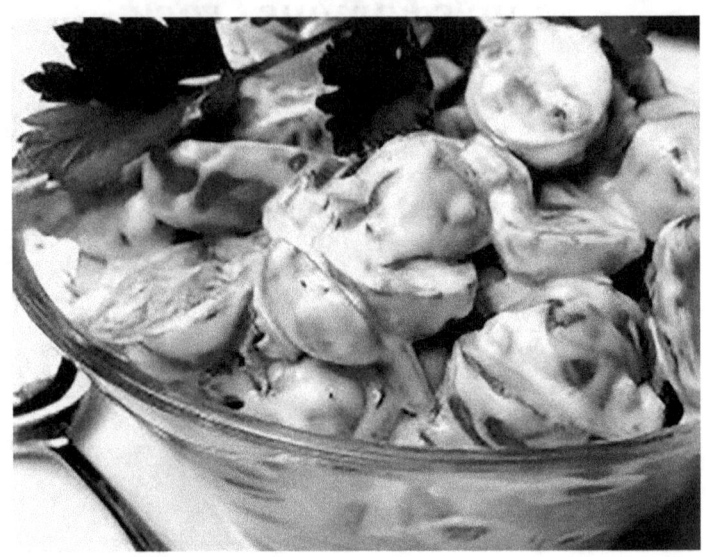

Ingredients

- 1/3 cup mayonnaise
- 2 teaspoons red wine vinegar
- 1 teaspoon Dijon mustard
- 1 pint cherry tomatoes, halved (I usually use grape tomatoes)
- 1/4 cup finely chopped red onion
- 2 tablespoons chopped fresh parsley
- Salt and pepper, to taste

Directions

1. Take mustard, mayonnaise, vinegar and whisk them together.

2. Then add onions. Then add tomatoes. Then add parsley.

3. Finally, toss and adjust the seasonings according to your taste and choice.

Parmesan Bow Ties

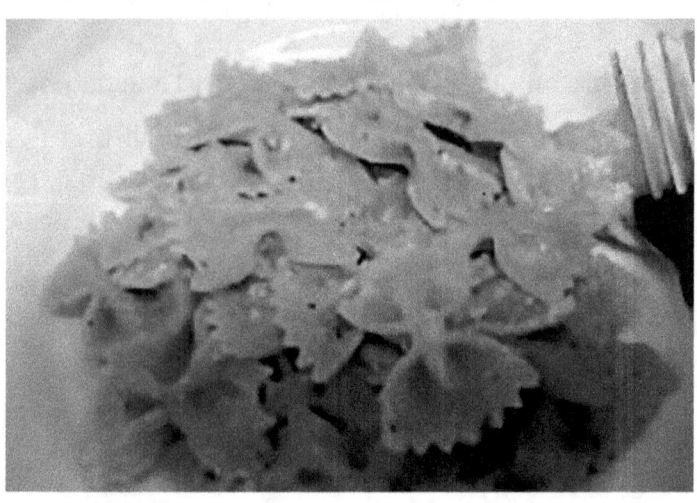

Ingredients

- 2 cups uncooked bow tie pasta
- 1/4 cup zesty Italian salad dressing
- 1/4 cup shredded parmesan cheese
- Salt and pepper
- 1 tablespoon minced parsley

Directions

1. First, prepare noodles as instructed on the package. Drain well.

2. Then shift to bowl. Take the rest of ingredients and add them. Toss well for the sake of coating.

Rice, Broccoli, & Cheese Casserole

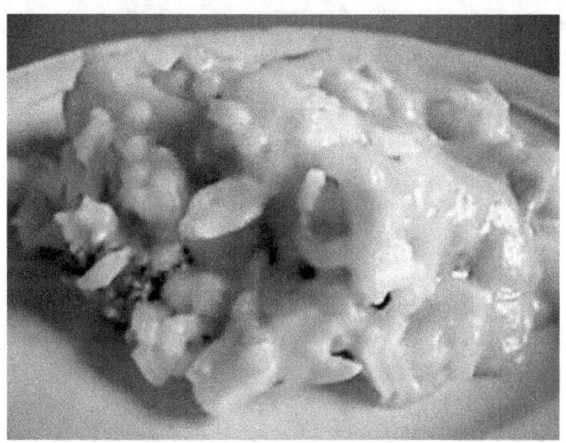

Ingredients

- 1 cup rice, cooked
- 1 cup milk
- 10 ounces frozen broccoli, cooked
- 1/2 lb. Velveeta cheese, cubed
- 1 small onion, diced
- 1 (10 3/4 ounce) cans cream of chicken soup
- 1 (4 ounce) cans mushrooms

Directions

1. Take all of the components/ingredients and blend them together in a big size casserole dish.

2. Then bake for FORTY FIVE min at 375 degrees Fahrenheit.

Curried Chickpeas & Kale

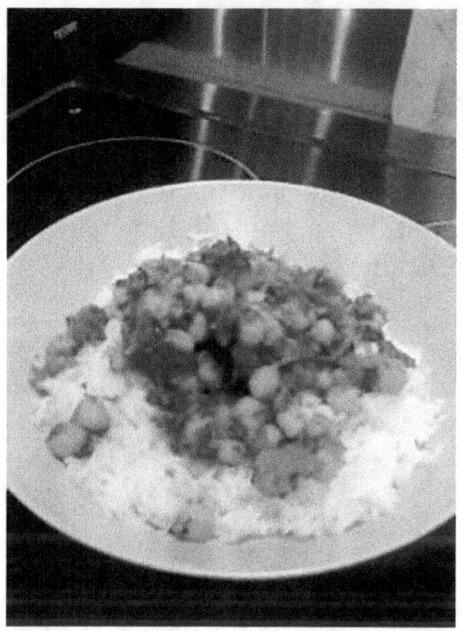

Ingredients

- 2 tablespoons vegetable oil
- 1 1/2 cups chopped onions
- 4 cloves garlic, minced
- 1/2 teaspoon cumin
- 3 cups chopped kale or 1 package frozen chopped spinach
- 1 1/2 tablespoons curry powder
- 1 teaspoon ground ginger
- 1 teaspoon ground coriander
- 1 1/2 cups vegetable broth

- 3 cups cooked chickpeas
- 1 cup chopped tomato
- 1/4 teaspoon salt

Directions

1. Take a crock pot and blend all of the above components/ingredients in this crockpot, and then cook on high temperature for FOUR hours.

Carrot Burgers

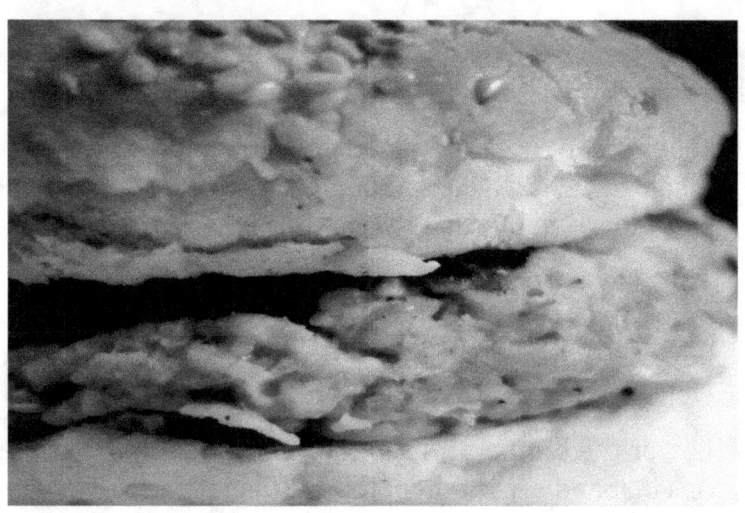

Ingredients

- 5 medium carrots, shredded (about 2 cups)
- 1 small yellow onion, finely chopped
- 3 tablespoons flour
- 2 tablespoons cornmeal
- 1 egg, lightly beaten
- 2 tablespoons milk (or half and half, or sour cream)
- 1 teaspoon dried dill weed
- 1/2 teaspoon sugar
- 1/2 teaspoon salt
- 1/4 teaspoon baking powder
- 1/8 teaspoon black pepper

- 2 tablespoons margarine
- 1 tablespoon olive oil

Directions

1. Take carrots, pepper, baking powder, onion, salt, flour, corn-meal, sugar, dill, egg and blend them together in moderate size bowl. Then form eight patties from the mixture.

2. Then shift to plate and use plastic wrap for covering it. Keep in refrigerator for sixty min, you can keep it up to twelve hours. Then take a heavy ten inch frying pan, heat oil as well as margarine in it for approximately one min.

3. Lower the temperature to medium. After this, put the patties in it and brown them for five to eight min on every side. Drain on plate that has been lined with paper towels.

Best Ever Black-Eyed Peas

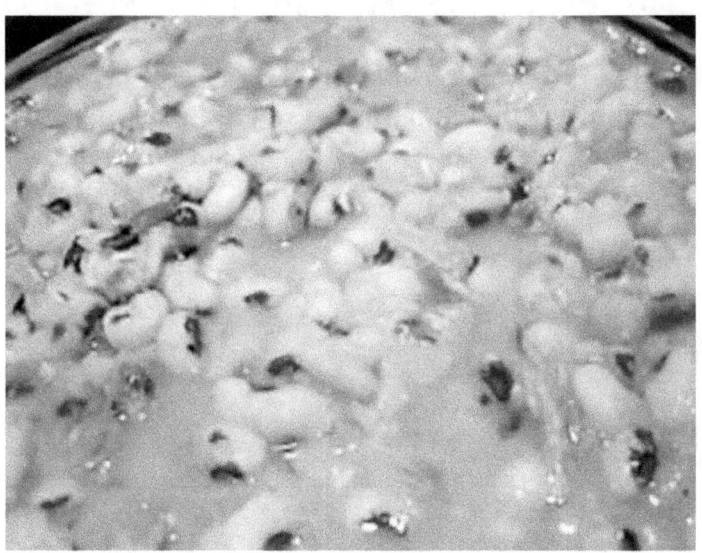

Ingredients

- 1 (16 ounce) packages dried black-eyed peas
- 6 cups water
- 1 medium onion, chopped
- 2 cloves garlic, minced
- 1 teaspoon salt
- 1/2 teaspoon black pepper
- 1 teaspoon sugar
- 1 ham hocks or 2 cups cooked ham, cut into small cubes
- 1 -2 jalapeno pepper, seeds removed and chopped

Directions

1. Take peas, sort them and then wash these peas. And then put them in large size Dutch oven.

2. Then take the rest of ingredients and add them. Heat to boiling.

3. Then lower the temperature and let it simmer for sixty to ninety min, covered or till peas get soften.

Potatoes Tapas in Garlic Mayonnaise (Potatoes Aioli)

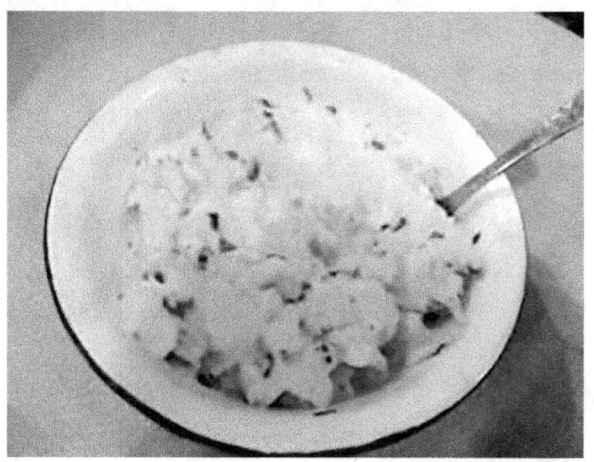

Ingredients

- 3/4 lb. salad potatoes
- 1/2 cup mayonnaise
- 3 garlic cloves, mashed to a paste or put through a garlic press
- 2 tablespoons parsley, minced
- Salt

Directions

1. Take potatoes and boil them in salted water till soften. Then peel these potatoes and chop them into chunks.
2. Then take a bowl, and mix in this bowl, parsley, garlic, mayonnaise.

3. Then right after this, take potatoes and fold them into sauce softly. Use salt as seasoning according to your taste. Serve deliciously.

Sweet Spicy Turnips

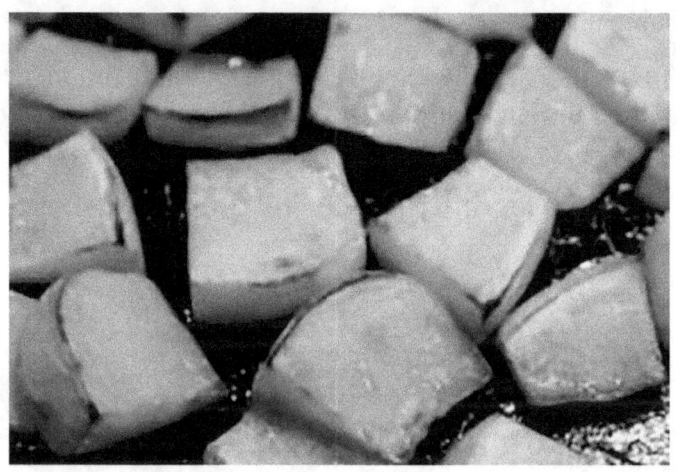

Ingredients

- 1 tablespoon brown sugar
- 2 teaspoons butter, melted
- 1/4 teaspoon salt
- 1/4 teaspoon crushed red pepper flakes
- 1/8 teaspoon ground ginger
- 1 dash ground allspice
- 3 turnips, peeled and each cut into 6 wedges (6 ounces each)
- Cooking spray

Directions

1. First of all, heat the oven to four hundred (400) degrees Fahrenheit.

2. After this, take the 1st SEVEN ingredients and mix them together in jelly roll pan that has been coated with cooking spray. Toss well.

3. Then bake for thirty five min till soften, mix after this, each ten min.

Buttered Baby Carrots and Sweet Peas

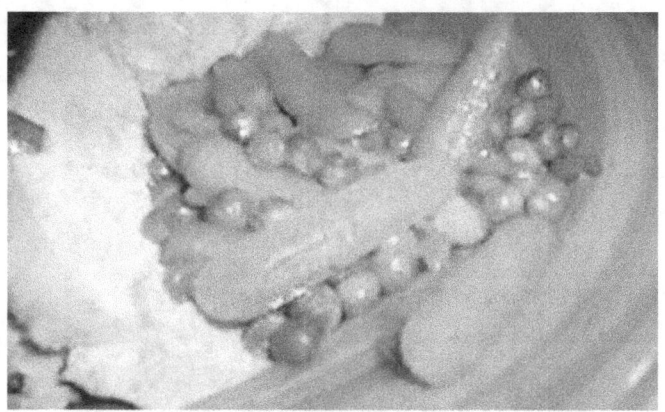

Ingredients

- 2 1/2 cups baby carrots, halved lengthwise
- 2 tablespoons butter
- 1 1/2 cups frozen peas
- 2 tablespoons water
- 1 teaspoon sugar
- Salt and pepper

Directions

1. Take carrots and quick fry them in butter in frying pan for five min.
2. Then mix in the rest of ingredients.
3. Then let it simmer for ten min, covered, or till veggies are ready and done.

Maroulosalata
(Classic Greek Lettuce Salad)

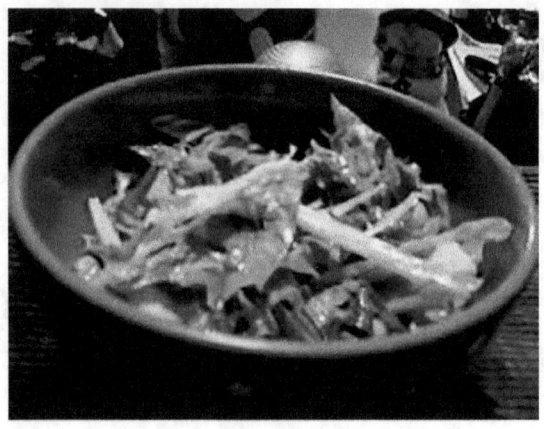

Ingredients

- 150 ml extra virgin olive oil
- 2 tablespoons white wine vinegar
- 1 romaine lettuce, shredded very finely
- 1 bunch spring onion, finely chopped, including the green parts
- 3 tablespoons finely chopped dill weed
- Sea salt, to taste
- Fresh ground pepper, to taste

Directions

1. Take oil, vinegar and blend them together in a bowl. Then take salt, pepper and add them according to your taste and choice.

2. Take the ingredients and mix them well. Toss well with the dressing. Serve right away.

Slow Cooker Stuffing

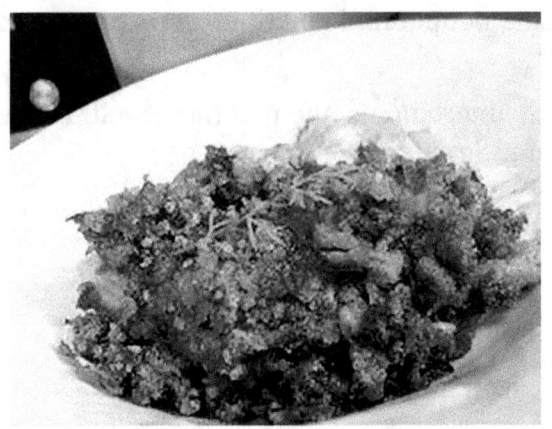

Ingredients

- 1 cup butter
- 2 cups chopped celery
- 1 cup chopped onion
- 1 teaspoon poultry seasoning
- 1 1/2 teaspoons sage leaves, crumbled
- 1/2 teaspoon pepper
- 1 1/2 teaspoons salt
- 1 teaspoon leaf thyme, crumbled
- 2 beaten eggs
- 4 cups chicken broth
- 12 cups dry breadcrumbs

Directions

1. Take a large size mixing bowl, mix in this bowl, broth, eggs, celery, spices, and butter.

2. Take bread crumbs and add them. Mix well.

3. Then prepare in slow cooker on high temperature for forty five min. lower the temperature for six hours.

Creamy Parmesan Leeks

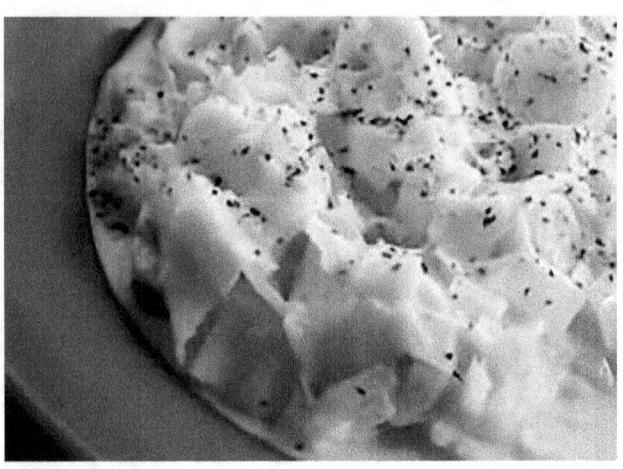

Ingredients

- 2 leeks, washed well and thinly sliced (white only)
- 3 tablespoons water
- 1 tablespoon butter
- 1/2 cup cream
- 1/4 cup parmesan cheese
- Cracked black pepper, plenty of it

Directions

1. Take a saucepan, put butter, water and leeks in this saucepan with fitting lid.

2. Heat to boiling, then lower the temperature and cook for approximately fifteen min.

3. Mix in cream. Then after this, fold in parmesan cheese. Delicious.

Big Texan Texas Caviar

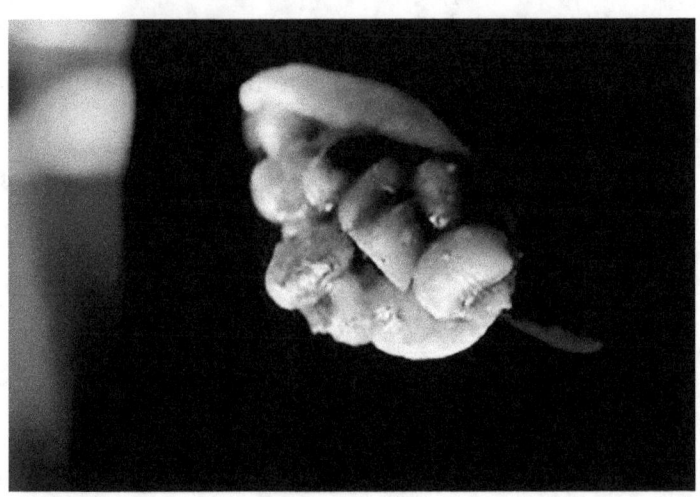

Ingredients

- 2 (16 ounce) cans black-eyed peas, drained
- 1 medium jalapeno, minced
- 1/4 small white onion, chopped
- 1/3 cup Italian dressing
- 1/2 green bell pepper, chopped
- 1 teaspoon seasoning salt
- 2 teaspoons chili powder
- 2 teaspoons ground cumin
- 1/3 teaspoon ground red pepper

Directions

1. Take black-eyed peas along with the rest of ingredients and blend them well.

2. Then let it chill.

3. You can serve this chilled recipe with corn chips.

Crab, Prosciutto & Green Onion Potato Cakes!

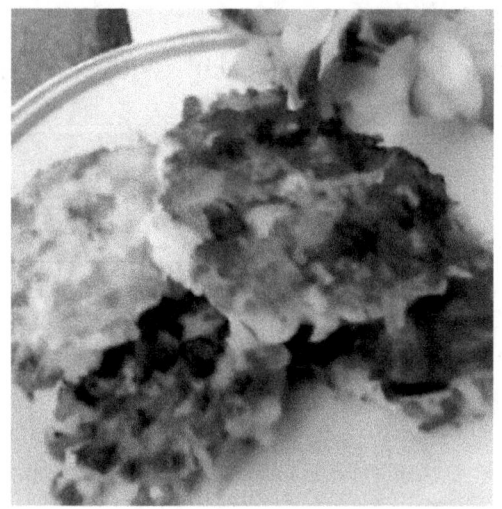

Ingredients

- 1 (20 ounce) bags Simply Potatoes Shredded Hash Browns
- 8 ounces lump crabmeat
- 4 ounces diced prosciutto
- 4 green onions, diced
- 3 eggs

Directions

1. First, take all of the above mentioned ingredients for this recipe and blend them well and make patties from this mixture.

2. Then fry on nonstick frying pan for six to seven min on each and every side till color changes to light brown.

3 STEP KID-FRIENDLY MEALS
Your Kids Time out Lunch

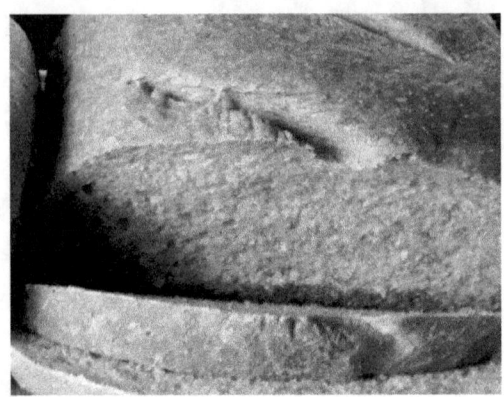

Ingredients

- 1 slice whole wheat bread
- 1 glass water

Directions

1. Take bread and place it on steel lunch tray. Then take glass of water and place it out.

Macaroni Salad

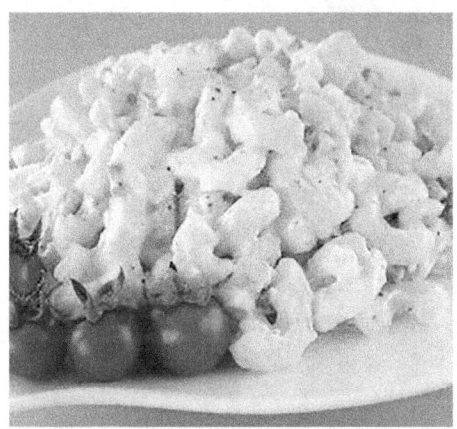

Ingredients

- Dressing
- 1 cup mayonnaise.
- 2 tablespoons vinegar
- 1 tablespoon mustard
- 1 teaspoon sugar
- 1 teaspoon salt
- 1/4 teaspoon pepper
- 1/2 lb. macaroni, cooked and drained
- 1 cup sliced celery
- 1/2 cup chopped green pepper
- 1/2 cup chopped red pepper
- 1/2 cup chopped green onion

Directions

1. Take the dressing ingredients and blend them together.
2. Then mix into the rest of ingredients.
3. Then cover it and let it chill.

Nutella Hot Chocolate

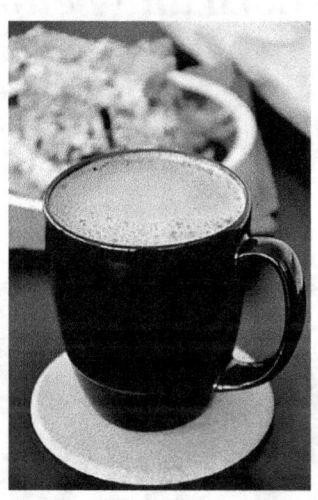

Ingredients

- 3 tablespoons Nutella
- 1 1/3 cups milk

Directions

1. Take Nutella® and ONE THIRD cup of milk and put them in small size saucepan over moderate temperature.

2. Blend well.

3. Then take the rest of milk and add them. Raise the temperature to moderately high temperature, whisk till frothy.

Halloween Party Treat (Candy Corn and Peanut Mix)

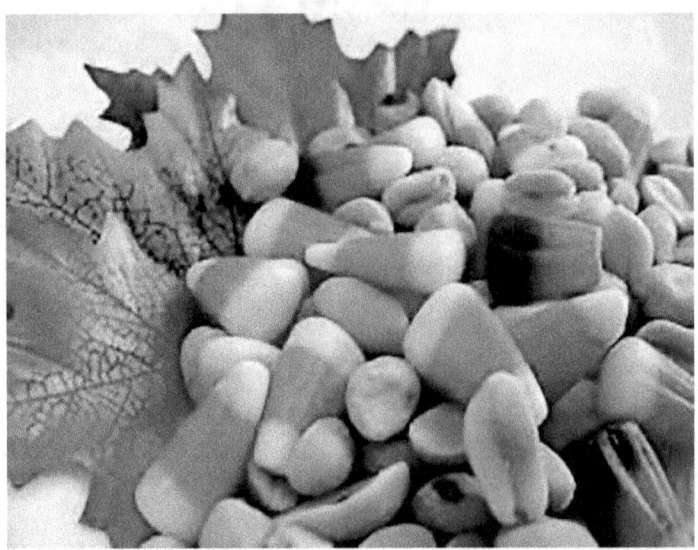

Ingredients

- 1 cup candy corn
- 1 cup salted peanuts

Directions

1. Take peanuts and mix them with candy corn together.
2. You can serve this recipe in a bowl.

Melt in Your Mouth Pumpkin Bread

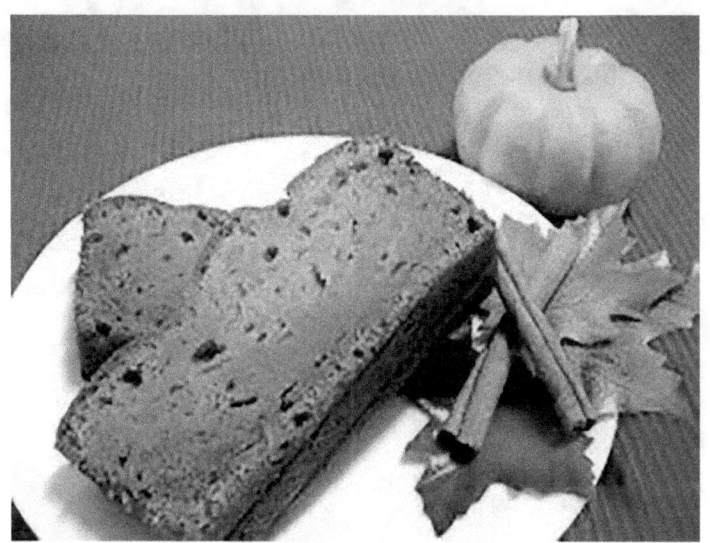

Ingredients

- 2/3 cup oil
- 2 large eggs
- 1 cup pumpkin
- 1 cup flour
- 1 cup sugar
- 1 (3 1/2 ounce) boxes instant coconut pudding mix
- 1/2 teaspoon salt
- 1/2 teaspoon baking soda
- 1/2 teaspoon cinnamon

Directions

1. Take pumpkin, eggs, oil and mix them together.
2. Take the rest of ingredients and combine them. Then after this, add to mixture of pumpkin.
3. Then bake for sixty min at 325 degrees Fahrenheit.

Breaded Ranch or Ranchero Chicken

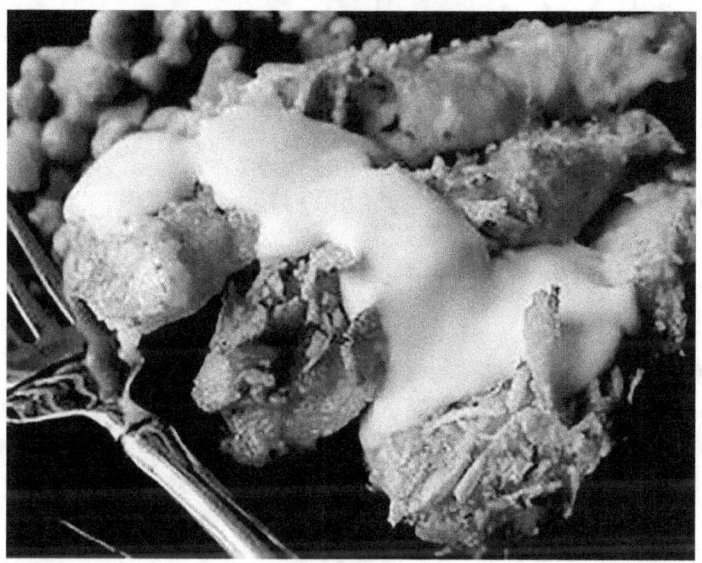

Ingredients

- 2 lbs. boneless skinless chicken breasts
- 3/4 cup parmesan cheese
- 3/4 cup crushed corn flakes
- 1 (1 ounce) envelope ranch dressing mix
- 1/2 cup melted butter or 1/2 cup melted margarine

Directions

1. Take a bowl and mix in this bowl, cheese, salad dressing mix and cereal.

2. Then take chicken and dip into melted butter and then after this, dip into the mixture you obtained above.

3. Then bake in a dish that has been greased, at 350 degrees Fahrenheit, covered, for approximately FORTY five min.

Sweet and Sour Meatballs

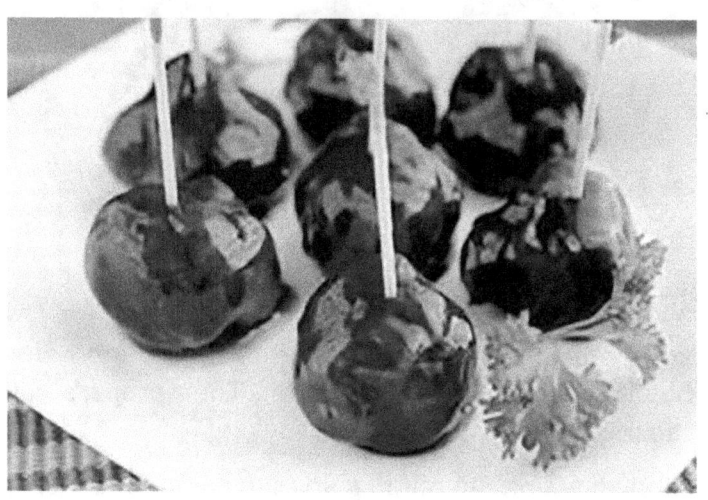

Ingredients

- For the meatballs
- 1 lb. ground beef
- Worcestershire sauce, to taste
- 3 tablespoons breadcrumbs
- Oregano, to taste
- 1 egg, slightly beaten
- Salt and pepper, to taste
- 1 clove garlic, minced
- 2 tablespoons vegetable oil
- For the sauce
- 1 tablespoon vegetable oil

- 1/2 cup onion, chopped
- 3/4 cup brown sugar, packed
- 2 tablespoons vinegar
- 1 teaspoon lemon juice
- 1 cup ketchup
- 2 tablespoons soya sauce

Directions

1. For preparing meatballs: take all of the ingredients and blend them together besides oil. Then prepare balls from the mixture.

2. After this, sauté in oil till golden in color and place them on paper towel for draining. Keep aside.

3. For preparing sauce: take medium size saucepan, sauté onion in oil till soften. Take rest of sauce ingredients and add them. Let it simmer for TWENTY min

4. Take meatballs and add them and cook them for SIXTY min on moderate temperature.

Layer Cookies
(Magic Layer Bars)

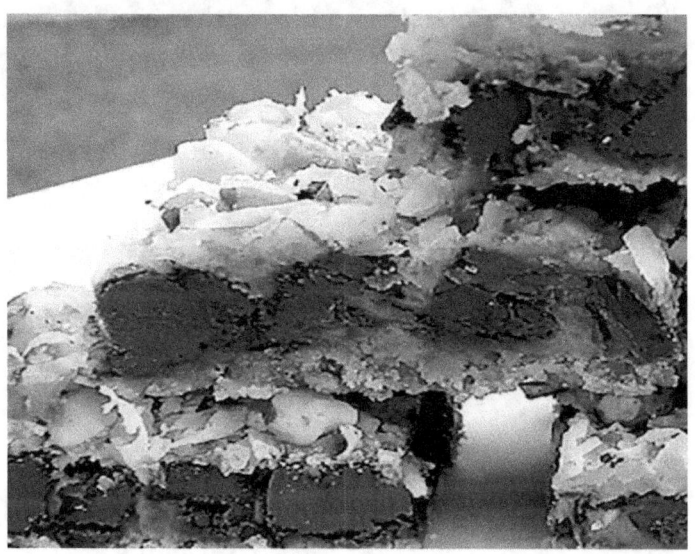

Ingredients

- 1/2 cup butter, melted
- 1 cup graham cracker, crushed to crumbs
- 1 cup flaked coconut
- 6 ounces chocolate chips (1 cup)
- 6 ounces butterscotch chips
- 1 (14 ounce) cans sweetened condensed milk (fat free works fine)
- 1 cup nuts

Directions

1. Take melted butter and put it in baking pan. Then take graham cracker crumbs and spread them over the top.

2. Take coconut and chips and layer them in the mentioned order. Take sweetened condensed milk and pour it all over. Use nuts as topping.

3. Finally, bake for TWENTY FIVE min, at 35o degrees Fahrenheit till color changes to lightly brown in color.

Butter Roasted Carrots

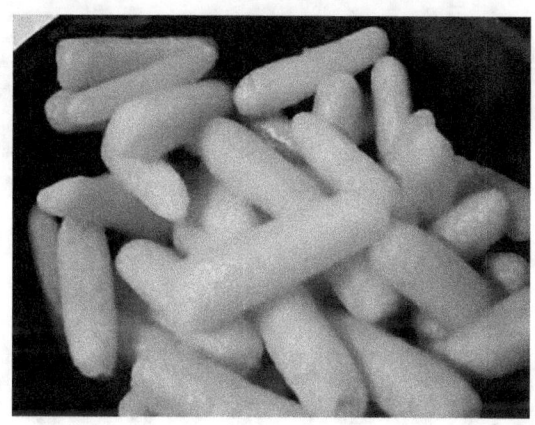

Ingredients

- 2 lbs. carrots
- 2 tablespoons butter

Directions

1. Take carrots, peel them and then chop them lengthwise. And then halve them.

2. Take carrots and place them in casserole dish. Take dollop butter and place over the top.

3. Then roast for sixty min at 350 degrees Fahrenheit, covered, mix after every TWENTY min.

Egg Salad Sandwich

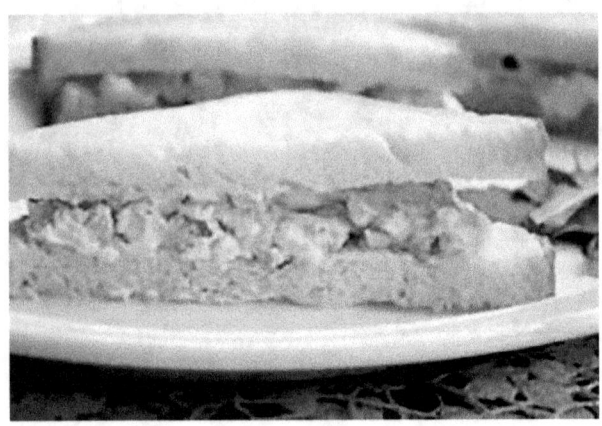

Ingredients

- 2 hard-boiled eggs
- 1 teaspoon minced onion
- 1/8 teaspoon celery seed
- 1/8 teaspoon Dijon mustard
- 1/4 cup shredded lettuce
- 2 tablespoons mayonnaise
- 2 slices bread
- Butter
- 1 dash salt and pepper

Directions

1. Take hard boiled eggs and finely chop them. Take onion, lettuce, mayo, Dijon, celery seed and add them. Blend well.

2. Take every bread slice and butter each one of the slices. Use egg mixture as topping.

3. Use salt and pepper as sprinkles. Then seal the sandwich and have fun.

3 STEP DESSERT MEALS
Vanilla Buttercream Frosting (From Sprinkles Cupcakes)

Ingredients

- 1 cup butter, softened
- 3 1/2 cups confectioners' sugar
- 1 teaspoon milk
- 1 teaspoon vanilla extract
- 1/8 teaspoon salt

Directions

1. First, take a bowl, and blend in this bowl, salt, sugar and butter. Mix till smooth.

2. Take vanilla, milk and add them. Beat for next THREE TO FIVE min or till creamy.

Bakery Buttercream Frosting/Icing

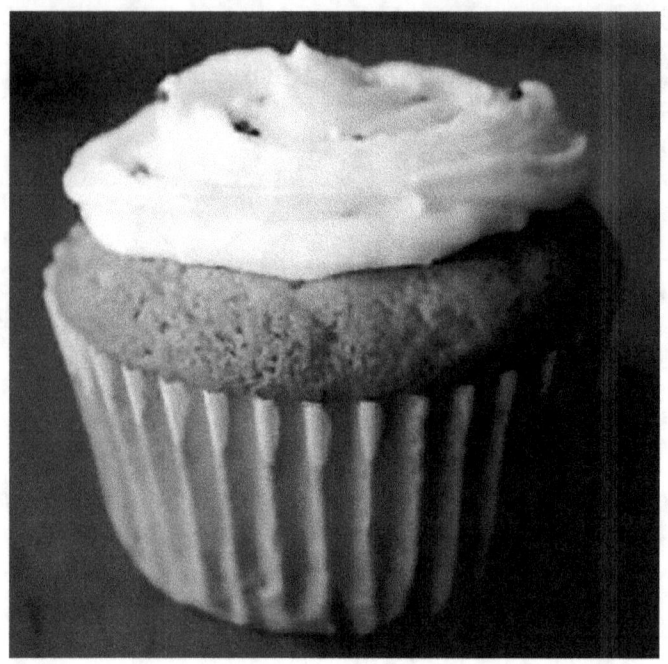

Ingredients

- 1/2 cup white Crisco shortening, softened
- 1/2 cup margarine, softened
- 4 -6 tablespoons 18% table cream
- 1 pinch salt
- 1/2 teaspoon almond extract
- 2 teaspoons vanilla
- 5 cups confectioners' sugar, sifted
- 2 -4 drops food coloring

Directions

1. First, take electric mixer and beat together shortening and margarine or butter with cream, salt almond extract and vanilla at moderate speed in large size bowl for approximately three min or till smooth enough.

2. Take the sifted confectioner sugar and add in. Beat until creamy and smooth.

3. Finally, use food coloring for achieving desired shade.

Butterfinger Pie

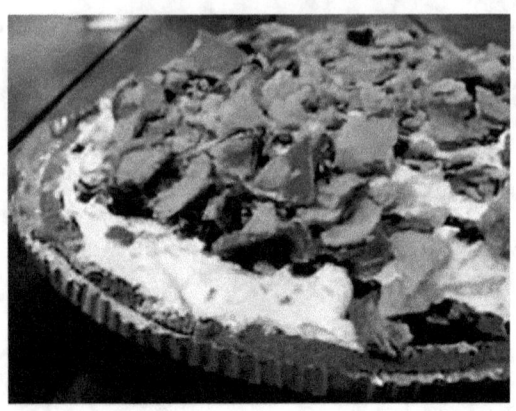

Ingredients

- 6 (2 1/8 ounce) Butterfinger® candy bars, crushed
- 1 (8 ounce) packages cream cheese
- 1 (12 ounce) cartons Cool Whip
- 1 graham cracker crust

Directions

1. Take the 1st components/ingredients and blend them together.
2. After this, take it and put in pie crust and chill.

Chocolate Syrup

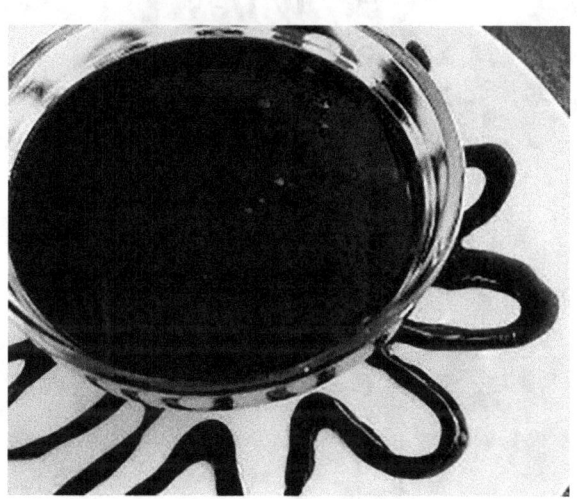

Ingredients

- 1 cup cocoa powder
- 1 1/2 cups sugar
- 1 dash salt
- 1 1/2 cups water
- 1 teaspoon vanilla extract

Directions

1. Take the ingredient and mix them together.
2. Then boil for two to five min, mix continuously, till sauce starts thicken.
3. You can keep this in fridge.

Intensely Chocolate Cocoa Brownies

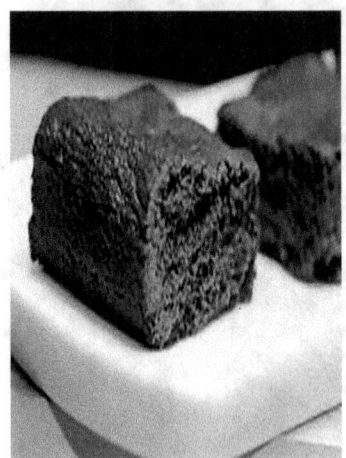

Ingredients

- 1/2 cup butter
- 1/2 cup cocoa
- 1 cup sugar
- 2 eggs
- 1 teaspoon vanilla
- 2/3 cup flour
- 1/2 teaspoon baking powder
- 1/4 teaspoon salt
- 1/2 cup walnuts (optional) or 1/2 cup chocolate chips (optional)

Directions

1. First, heat the oven to THREE HUNDRED 50 (350) degrees Fahrenheit.

2. Take a saucepan and melt butter in it. Then take it away from heat. Take cocoa and mix in well. Take vanilla, sugar, eggs and add them as well. Blend till smooth.

3. Take salt, baking powder, flour and add them. Blend well. Take either choc chips or walnuts and add it.

4. Take EIGHT inch pan and pour into it and bake for FIFTEEN TO TWENTY min. then let it cool

Quick-N-Easy
Fruit Dip

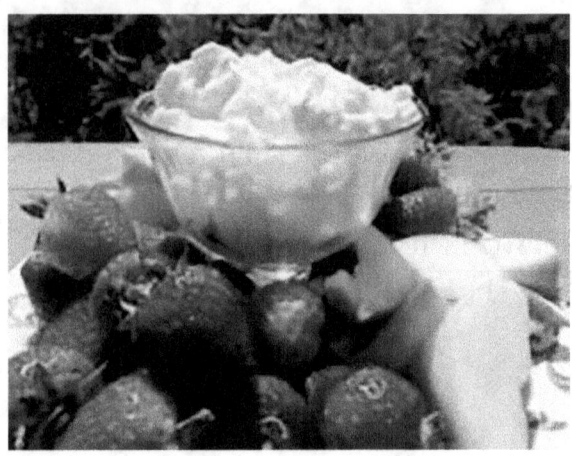

Ingredients

- 8 ounces Philadelphia Cream Cheese
- 7 ounces marshmallow creme
- Cantaloupe or honeydews or pineapple or strawberries or watermelon, cubed

Directions

1. First, take marshmallow crème and cream cheese and blend them together till blended and smooth.
2. Once ready, you can serve this with fruit.

Monster Cookies

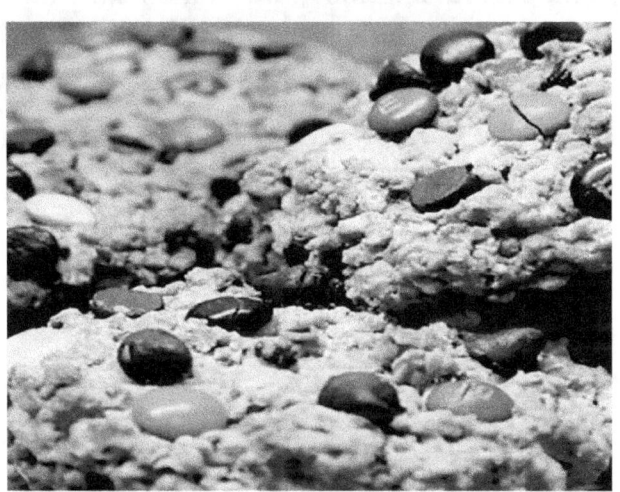

Ingredients

- 1 cup brown sugar
- 1 cup sugar
- 1/2 cup margarine, softened
- 3 eggs
- 1 teaspoon vanilla
- 1 teaspoon light syrup (Karo or pancake)
- 1 1/2 cups peanut butter
- 2 teaspoons baking soda
- 4 1/2 cups oatmeal
- 1 cup semi-sweet chocolate chips
- 4 ounces M&M's plain chocolate candy or 4 ounces M&M's peanut chocolate candies

Directions

1. Take the ingredients above and combine them well till well mixed.

2. Then after this, drop by teaspoonful on cookie sheet that is ungreased.

3. Finally, bake for FIFTEEN min at 350 degrees Fahrenheit.

Crock Pot Candy

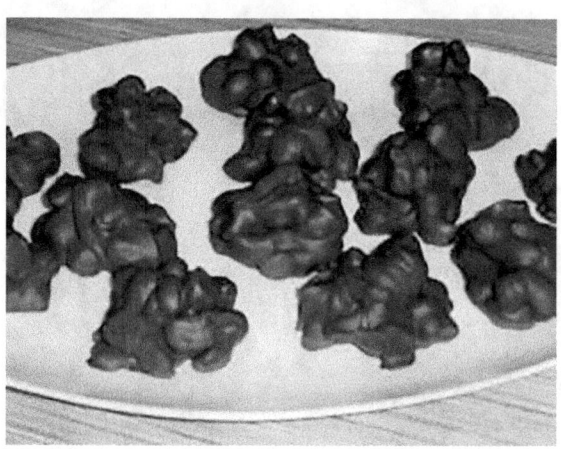

Ingredients

- 1 (16 ounce) packages dry roasted salted peanuts
- 1 (16 ounce) packages unsalted dry roasted peanuts
- 1 (12 ounce) packages semi-sweet chocolate bits
- 1 (4 ounce) German chocolate bars
- 32 ounces white almond bark

Directions

1. Take peanuts and place them in crockpot's bottom. Take the rest of ingredients and add them as well.

2. Then cook on low temperature for 90 to 120 min.

3. Then finally, take rounded spoonfuls and place them onto wax paper and let it cool.

Carrot Cake

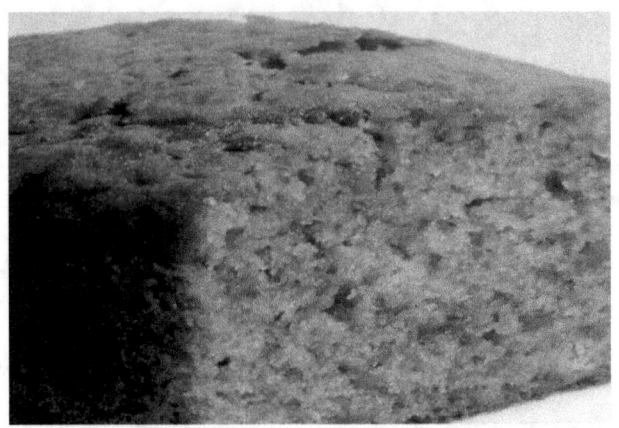

Ingredients

- 1 1/2 cups oil
- 3 eggs
- 2 cups sugar
- 2 1/2 cups flour
- 2 cups grated raw carrots
- 2 teaspoons baking soda
- 2 teaspoons cinnamon
- 1 (20 ounce) cans crushed pineapple
- 1 cup chopped nuts (I use walnuts)
- 1 teaspoon salt
- Icing
- 1 (8 ounce) packages cream cheese
- 1 tablespoon margarine

- 1 lb. powdered sugar
- 1 teaspoon vanilla
- 1 -2 teaspoon milk, to thin
- 1 dash salt

Directions

1. First, take all of the cake components/ingredients and blend them together.
2. Bake for 50 min at 350 degrees Fahrenheit in baking pan.
3. After this, take all of the icing ingredients and combine them till well mixed and cover the cake.

Cinnamon Oranges

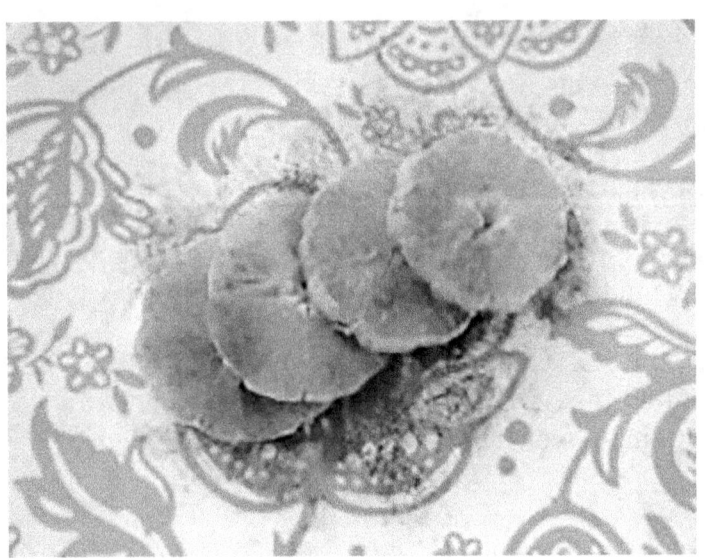

Ingredients

- 2 oranges, the sweetest you can find
- 1 apple, sliced (optional)
- 1 tablespoon cinnamon

Directions

1. Take oranges and peel them, after this, crosswise slice them into round shapes and then organize them on a plate.
2. If you like, take a couple of slices of apple and add them too.
3. After this, use cinnamon for light dusting and serve right away.

Peanut Butter Frosting

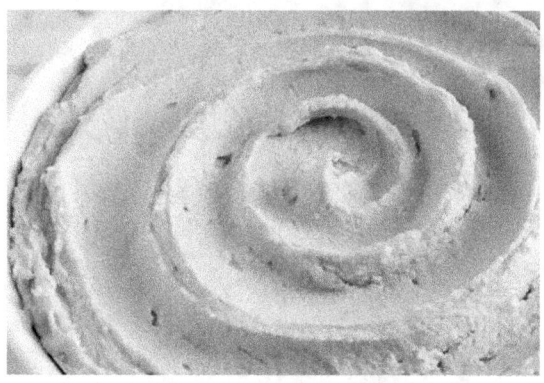

Ingredients

- 1/2 cup peanut butter, smooth
- 5 tablespoons margarine, softened
- 1 cup powdered sugar (or more, to taste)
- 1 -3 tablespoon milk (only if needed to thin) (optional)

Directions

1. Take the butter and beat them together with the help of electric mixer. Then take sugar and add it.
2. You can add a little bit of milk of it is very thick.

Rhubarb Crisp

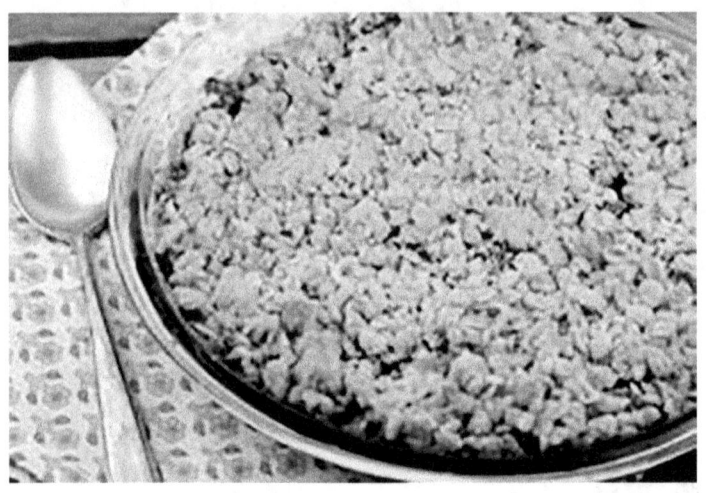

Ingredients

- 4 cups rhubarb, cut into 3/4 " pieces
- 1 cup sugar
- 1/4 cup flour
- 1/2 teaspoon cinnamon
- 1 cup flour
- 1 cup brown sugar
- 1/2 cup rolled oats
- 1/2 cup melted butter

Directions

1. First, take cinnamon, rhubarb, flour and sugar AND COM-BINE THEM TOGETHER and put in glass baking dish.

2. Then take melted butter, rolled oats, brown sugar, and flour and combine them together.

3. Take streusel and sprinkle it all over the rhubarb mixture. Finally, bake FOR THIRTY FIVE min at THREE HUNDRED SEVENTY FIVE (375) degrees Fahrenheit.

Dreamsicle Jell-O Salad

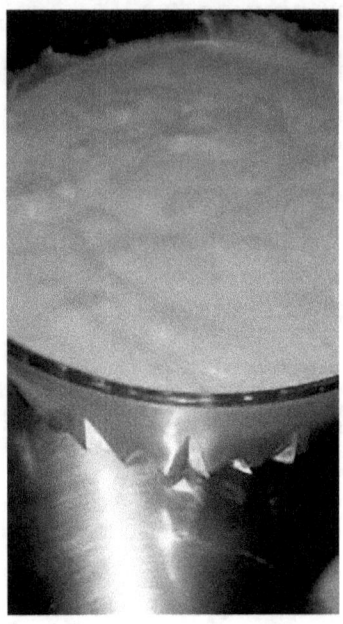

Ingredients

- 2 (3 ounce) packages instant vanilla pudding
- 1 (3 ounce) packages orange Jell-O®
- 1 1/2 cups boiling water
- 1 (22 ounce) cans mandarin oranges (with juice)
- 1 (16 ounce) containers Cool Whip

Directions

1. Take boiling water, jello, pudding and combine them together till thoroughly dissolved.

2. Take mandarin oranges along with juice and add them.

3. Finally, fold in cool whip.

Apple or Pear Crisp for One

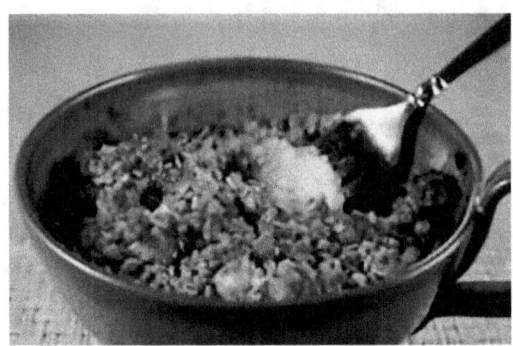

Ingredients

- 1 apples or 1 pear, peeled and thinly sliced
- 2 tablespoons brown sugar
- 2 tablespoons quick-cooking oats
- 1 tablespoon flour
- 1/8 teaspoon cinnamon
- 1 tablespoon butter

Directions

1. Take fruit and put it in small size baking dish.
2. Then take a separate bowl, combine in this bowl, the rest of ingredients and then sprinkle over fruit.
3. Finally, bake for TWENTY FIVE Min at 375 degrees Fahrenheit.

One Bowl Gluten Free Chocolate Cake

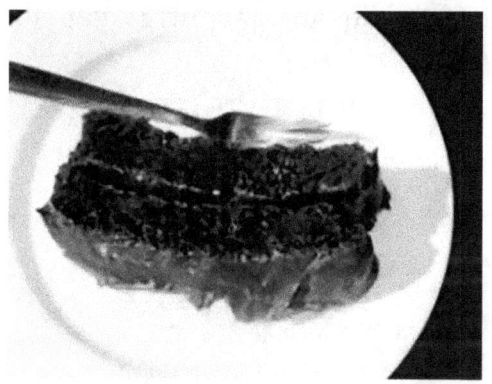

Ingredients

- 1 1/2 cups gluten-free flour
- 1/2 cup cocoa
- 1 cup sugar
- 1/2 teaspoon salt
- 2 teaspoons baking soda
- 3/4 teaspoon guar gum or 3/4 teaspoon xanthan gum
- 5 tablespoons cooking oil
- 1 tablespoon vinegar
- 1 teaspoon pure vanilla extract
- 1 egg
- 1 cup water

Directions

1. Take all of the dry components/ingredients and blend them in a bowl.

2. Take all of the liquid components/ingredients and blend them well.

3. Then bake for THIRTY TO THIRTY FIVE Min at 35o degrees Fahrenheit, in greased as well as floured square shape pan.

3 STEP ONE DISH MEALS
Polish Sausage Dinner

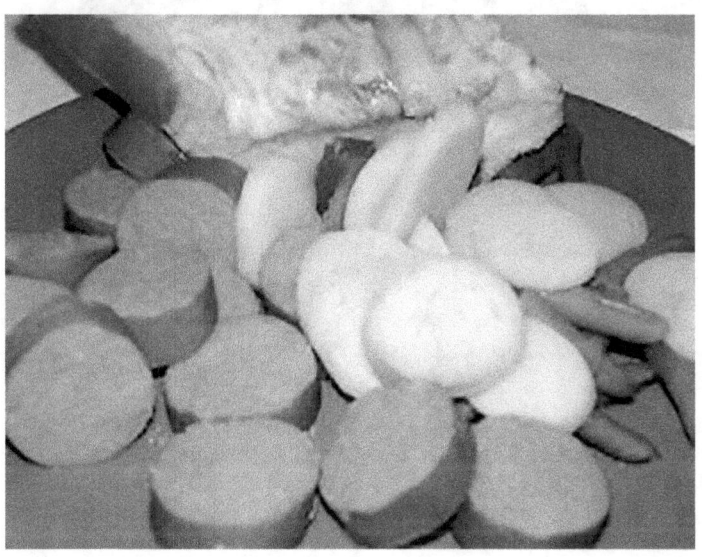

Ingredients

- 1 (14 ounce) packages beef Polish sausage
- 1 (14 ounce) cans sliced potatoes
- 1 (14 ounce) cans cut green beans

Directions

1. Take all of the ingredients and put them in skillet and heat it till ready and done, it takes ten to fifteen min.

Moroccan Ground Beef Kebab / Skewers

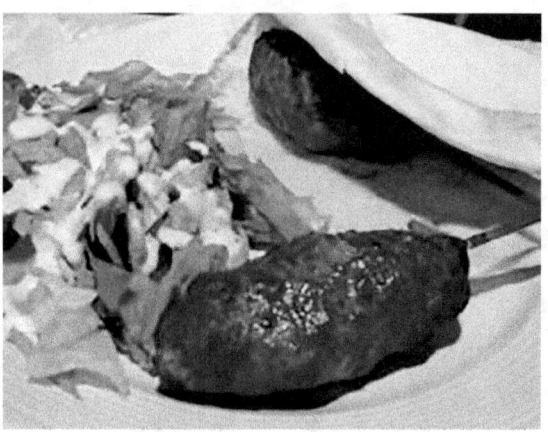

Ingredients

- 2 lbs. ground beef
- 1/2 medium onion, grated
- 2 garlic cloves, minced
- 1 tablespoon fresh parsley, finely chopped
- 1 tablespoon fresh cilantro, finely chopped
- 1 teaspoon paprika
- 1 teaspoon cumin
- 1/2 teaspoon salt
- 1/2 teaspoon black pepper
- 1/2-1 teaspoon cayenne pepper
- 1/2 teaspoon ras el hanout spice mix, Ras El Hanout - Moroccan Spice Mix

Directions

1. Take a large size bowl and combine in this bowl, spices, cilantro, parsley, onion and beef. And then keep in refrigerator for SIXTY min.

2. Then take small quantity of meat mixture and pack around the skewers.

3. Finally, grill over charcoal, turn them and cook completely.

4. You can serve this recipe with Authentic Moroccan Bread.

Diabetic Shrimp Scampi

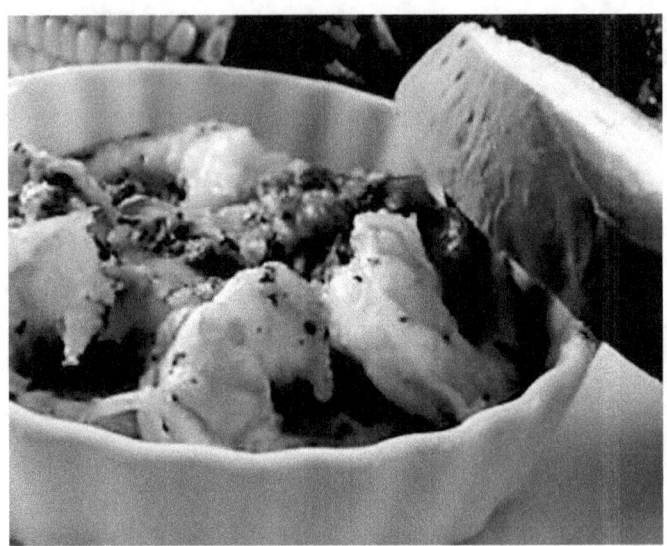

Ingredients

1. 1 tablespoon butter
2. 2 tablespoons olive oil
3. 4 garlic cloves, finely chopped
4. 11 -15 medium shrimp, peeled and deveined
5. 1/4 cup dry white wine
6. 1 tablespoon fresh lemon juice
7. 1/2 teaspoon salt
8. 1/8 teaspoon black pepper
9. 1 tablespoon seasoned dry bread crumb
10. 2 tablespoons fresh parsley, chopped

Directions

1. Take butter and oil and heat them in large size nonstick frying pan over high temperature. Then add garlic. Lower the temperature and cook for ONE min, mix.

2. Take shrimp and add it and cook for two min, mix from time to time. Take wine, lemon juice and add them.

3. Then take salt and pepper and add them. Cook for two min or till shrimp are heated and cooked through. Then mix in breadcrumbs. Then mix in parsley.

Kielbasa-Bean Slow Cooker Soup

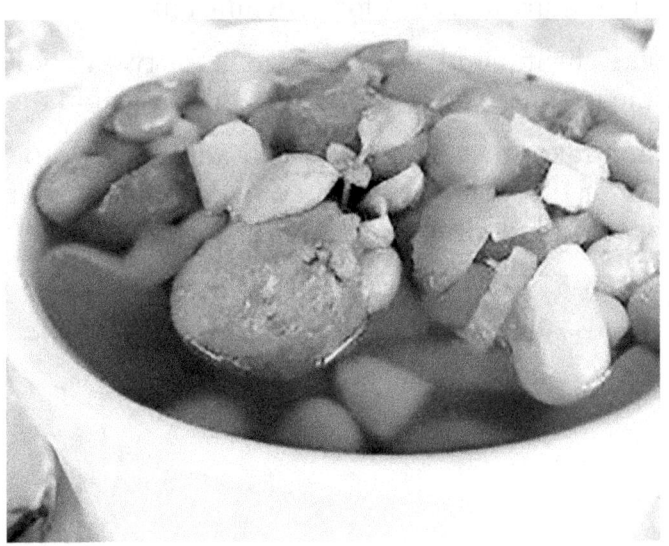

Ingredients

- 58 ounces fat-free chicken broth, four 14. 5 oz. cans
- 16 ounces low-fat smoked sausage
- 15 ounces canned pinto beans, rinsed and drained
- 15 ounces canned black beans, rinsed and drained
- 4 medium carrots, chopped
- 3 stalks celery, chopped
- 1 large onion, chopped
- 1 teaspoon thyme
- 14 1/2 ounces diced tomatoes, undrained

Directions

1. Take all of the components/ingredients and blend them well, in six quart slow cooker.

2. Then cook on low temperature, covered, for a minimum of six hours or till veggies get soften.

3. Mix in tomatoes. Then cook over high temperature, covered, for approximately fifteen min extra.

Goat Cheese and Spinach Turkey Burgers

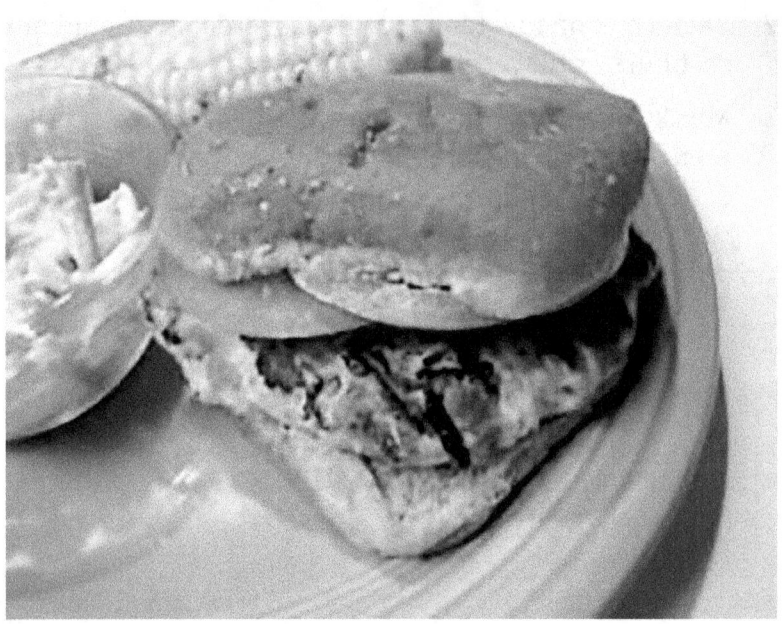

Ingredients

- 1 1/2 lbs. ground turkey breast
- 1 cup frozen chopped spinach, thawed and drained
- 2 tablespoons goat cheese, crumbled

Directions

1. First of all, heat the oven broiler.

2. Then take a medium size bowl, mix together in this bowl, goat cheese, spinach, ground turkey. Make FOUR patties from the mixture.

3. After this, organize these patties on broiler pan and put in the center of oven for FIFTEEN min or till ready and done.

Easy One-Dish Quinoa and Tuna

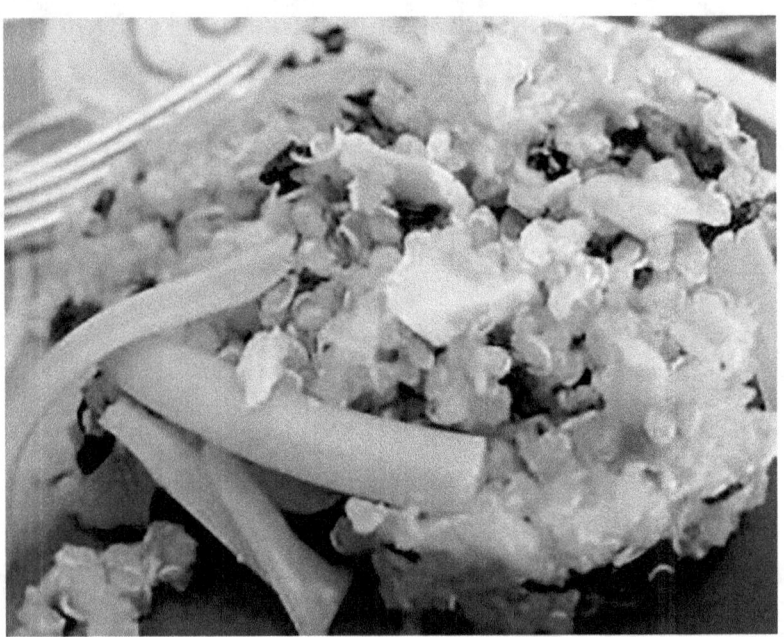

Ingredients

- 1 1/2 cups quinoa
- 3 cups chicken broth
- 3/4 cup frozen spinach
- 1/3 onion, diced
- 1 teaspoon minced garlic (depending on how garlicky you like it!)
- 1/2 teaspoon Italian seasoning
- Salt (to taste)

- 6 ounces tuna
- 1/2 cup cheese (optional)

Directions

1. Take all of the ingredients and mix them in medium size saucepan besides cheese and tuna.

2. Use lid for coving the saucepan and heat to boiling. Lower the temperature and let it simmer for FIFTEEN min till liquid is assimilated.

3. Take away from heat. Take cheese as well as tuna and add them.

Marilyn's Mac and Cheese with Tomatoes

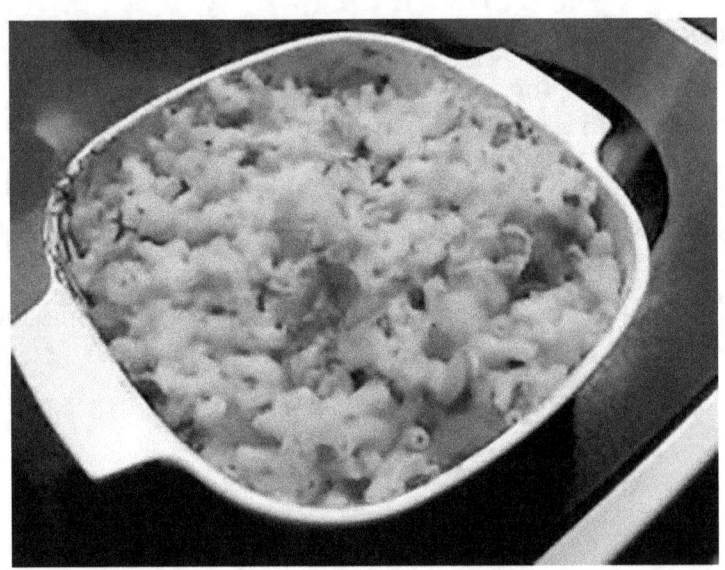

Ingredients

- 2 cups shell macaroni
- 1/4 cup cheddar cheese, grated
- 1/4 cup monterey jack cheese, grated
- 1/4 cup provolone cheese, grated (or use Mexican cheese blend for all three cheeses)
- 1/2 cup sour cream
- 1 (15 ounce) cans diced stewed tomatoes, drained
- 1 tablespoon unsalted butter
- 2 teaspoons fresh oregano

Directions

1. First of all, heat the oven to THREE HUNDRED 50 (350) degrees Fahrenheit. Cook macaroni as instructed on the package. Then drain well and shift to ONE quart casserole dish.

2. Then mix in rest of ingredients. Then bake for approximately THIRTY min till bubbly.

Crock Pot Chuck Roast

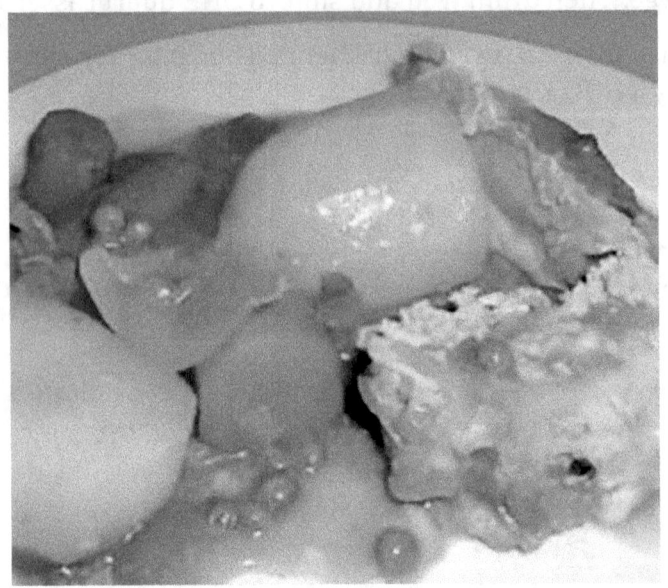

Ingredients

- 4 lbs. boneless chuck roast, cut up in pieces
- 1 (10 1/2 ounce) cans cream of mushroom soup
- 1/4 cup A-1 Steak Sauce
- 1 (1 1/4 ounce) packages onion soup mix
- 3/4 cup water

Directions

1. Take all of the ingredients and place them in crockpot.
2. Then cook for low temperature for EIGHT hours.

Tangy Greek Chicken Soup (Crock Pot or Not)

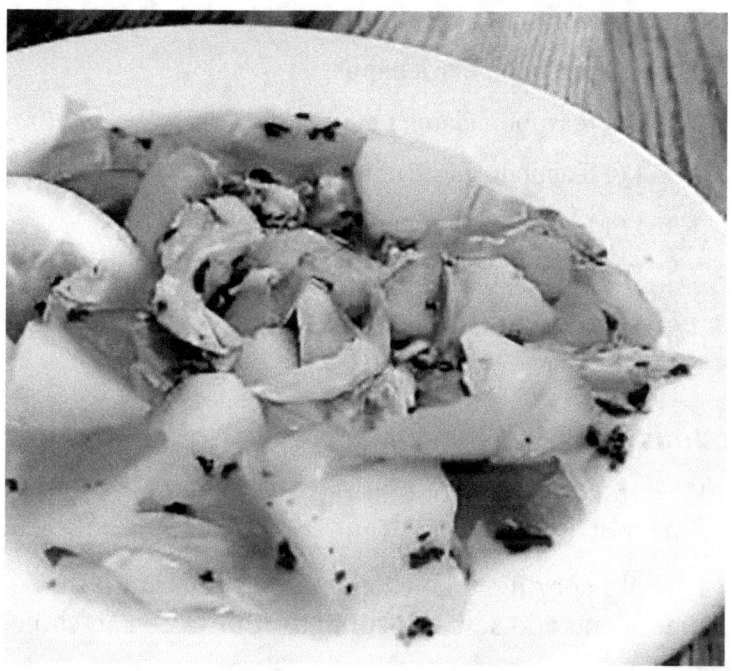

Ingredients

- 2 boneless skinless chicken breasts
- 3 large potatoes, roughly diced
- 18 baby carrots, sliced
- 1 onion, coarsely chopped
- 3 garlic cloves, minced
- 1 cup marinated artichoke hearts, drained, coarsely chopped
- 1 lemon, juice of

- 2 (15 ounce) cans chicken broth
- 1 cup white wine
- 1/4 cup white wine vinegar
- 2 tablespoons fresh oregano or 1 tablespoon dried oregano
- 1/8-1/4 teaspoon black pepper
- 1/8-1/4 teaspoon lemon pepper
- 1/8-1/4 teaspoon garlic powder
- 1/8-1/4 teaspoon onion powder
- 1/8-1/4 teaspoon ground coriander
- 1/8-1/4 teaspoon sugar

Directions

1. First, take a crockpot and put all of the ingredients in this crockpot. Cook for SIXTY min on high temperature.
2. Prior to serving, take chicken and break it up into eatable pieces and add salt according to your taste and choice.

Stewed Tomatoes and Garbanzo Beans

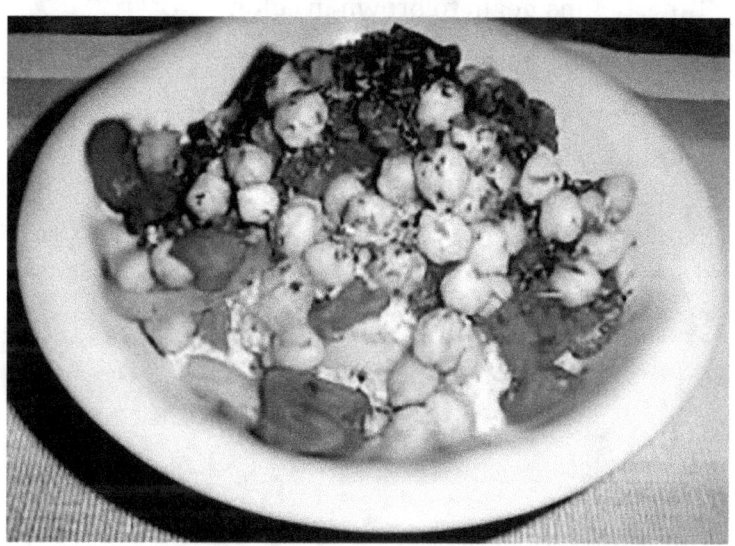

Ingredients

- 1 tablespoon olive oil
- 1 1/2 cups onions, sliced in half lengthwise, and then thinly sliced
- 2 garlic cloves, minced
- 2 (16 ounce) cans garbanzo beans, drained
- 1 (28 ounce) cans whole tomatoes, do not drain
- 1/4 teaspoon salt (to taste)
- 1/8 teaspoon fresh ground black pepper (to taste)

Directions

1. Take medium size saucepan and heat oil in it. Quick fry garlic as well onion for FIVE TO SEVE min, mix from time to time, onions begin to brown in color.

2. Take rest of ingredients and add them.

3. Then let it simmer for EIGHT TO TEN min, covered, mix from time to time, take away the cover. Serve deliciously.

Dijon Chicken Fettuccine

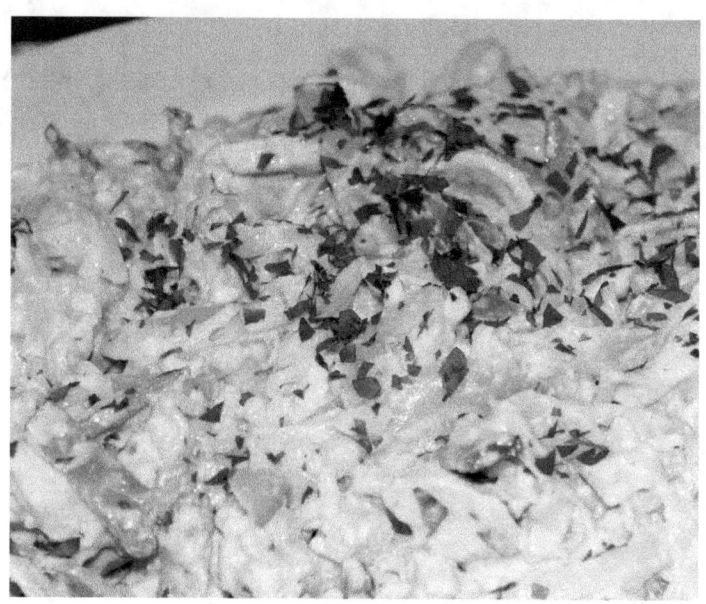

Ingredients

- 1 (9 ounce) packages spinach fettuccine
- 3/4 cup heavy cream
- 2 tablespoons Dijon mustard
- 1 1/2 cups diced cooked chicken
- 1/4 cup chopped roasted red pepper (optional)

Directions

1. Take fettuccine and cook it as instructed on the package. Drain and bring back the pasta to pot.

2. Take cream, mustard add to pasta in pot. Cook over moderate temperature for approximately two min, blend well.

3. Take chicken, red peppers add them.

Easy Chicken Pot Pie

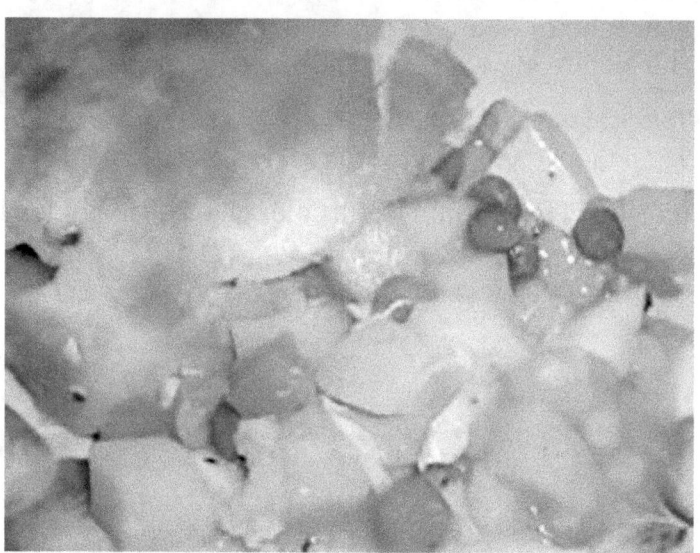

Ingredients

- 1 (16 ounce) packages frozen mixed vegetables, thawed
- 1 1/2 cups cut up cooked chicken
- 1 (10 3/4 ounce) cans condensed cream of chicken soup
- 1 cup original Bisquick® baking mix
- 1/2 cup milk
- 1 egg

Directions

1. First of all, heat the oven to FOUR HUNDRED (4oo) degrees Fahrenheit. Take veggies and mix them with soup and chicken in ungreased TWO QUART casserole.

2. Take small size bowl, and mix in the rest of ingredients in it. Then take it and pour onto casserole.

3. Bake for THIRTY min or till color changes to golden brown.

Quickie Mexican Pizza for One

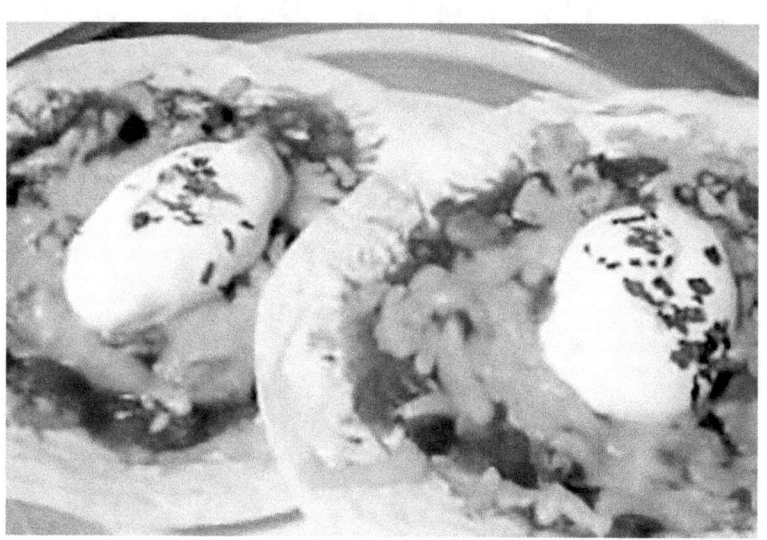

Ingredients

- 1 (6 inch) flour tortillas
- 1/4 cup salsa
- 1/4 cup canned black beans or 1/4 cup cooked black beans
- 1/4 cup shredded cheddar cheese (2% fat is fine) or 1/4 cup Mexican blend cheese
- 2 tablespoons diced green chilies

Directions

1. Take toppings and spread them on tortilla in the above given order.

2. Then bake for TEN min at 325 degrees Fahrenheit.

HEALTHY SNACKS FOR WORK

DIRT CHEAP & DELICIOUS, QUICK-TO-FIX HEALTHY WORK SNACKS

Introduction

I want to thank you and congratulate you for purchasing the book, "Healthy Snacks for Work".

There are multiple ways to eat and live healthy in this world today. It seems every time you turn around someone or something is coming to you in the media espousing a new idea on what to put to put your body and what to do to your body. But, many times these leave you wanting more, and never satisfying and please excuse the pun, not satisfied for what you came for.

Well, that's why this book was brought to you today. This is why you're reading this manuscript. You had a choice to find something new to help you to see your body in a new light, to break through the clutter and bring you something that will hopefully improve your life for the better and give you rock solid advice, and a new perspective.

This book contains proven steps and strategies on how to finally break through the mental barriers that you have with eating right at work, but also practical advice on how to avoid hunger pains that are so common with dips in blood sugar, coming at comes with not fueling your body right the first time

Thanks again for purchasing this book, I hope you enjoy it!

CHAPTER 1

Diet, Snacking, And Nutrition

People need food to survive. However, it is important that people eat a well-balanced diet. One of the main foundations of good health is healthy eating. This includes ingesting high-quality carbohydrates, proteins, healthy fats, minerals, vitamins, and water. The intake of processed foods, alcohol, and saturated fats should be minimized, or better yet, eliminated completely. By eating healthy, the body is able to maintain functions every day, promote the optimal body weight of a person, and help in preventing disease.

The nutrients that people get from the food can really help with their daily activities, they also help safeguard the body from the damage that the environment could bring about. Proteins are helpful in repairing injured tissues in the body, as well as promoting a good and healthy immune system. Fats and carbohydrates are essential for providing energy to the body. Minerals and vitamins support the different body processes. Certain vitamins (A, C, and E) act to protect the cells to drive out toxins. The B vitamins help to take out the energy from the food you ingest. Potassium and sodium help the nerves to transmit signals better, while phosphorus and calcium help strengthen bones. When one does not have a healthy diet, the different processes that need these elements will be disrupted.

In terms of eating healthy, quality and quantity both matters. Everyone must know that it is important to know how much food is enough for their bodies. By consuming roughly the same number of calories that the body is able to burn, one's weight will then stay the same over time. However, when people eat more food than what their body can metabolize effectively, weight gain will ensue. The extra calories are turned by the body into fat, and the more fat tissue that one has in the body, the higher the risk of developing health problems like hypertension, diabetes, heart disease, and cancer. Coming up with a meal plan that is healthy in all aspects will not only make one feel a lot better, but it will also help prolong one's life.

As mentioned in the previous paragraph, when people consume more calories than what their bodies can burn, they become overweight, or worse, obese. Obesity is not the only condition that is nutrition-related. Too little or too much of various nutrients can also be linked to health issues. For example, when people do not have enough calcium in the diet, they may be more prone to developing osteoporosis. Too much saturated fat in the diet can predispose a person to cardiovascular disease. When there are not enough fruits and vegetables in the diet, there is a higher risk of developing cancer. It helps to consume foods that come from a variety of food groups, even snacks.

If you aren't used to a healthy diet, you can make gradual changes to your diet at first. These small steps, such as changing your snacks for healthier alternatives, can help you eat healthier in the long run. For example, you can substitute your daily sugary soda for water or fresh juice. You can also switch from full-fat dairy products to low-fat. By making better choices for your meals, you are actually decreasing your risk of developing various diseases, and you are also improving your health. Healthier alternatives for snacks will go a long way to improving your overall health.

CHAPTER 2

How To Get Started On Healthy Eating And Snacking

When it comes to healthy eating, everything starts with learning new methods to eat, like incorporating more fresh vegetables, fruits, and whole grains into the diet. Foods that contain a lot of salt, sugar, and fat should be cut, not only during meal times, but for snacks, too. Transitioning to healthy eating also includes having to learn about moderation, balance, and variety.

Always practice moderation.

Remember that too much and too little of something is not good, so eat in moderation. All types of food, when taken in moderation, are acceptable for healthy eating; and fortunately, this also includes sweets.

A balanced meal should be your goal.

Be sure to listen to your body when you eat. Include foods from each of the food groups on most days, such as vegetables, fruits, grains, protein foods, and dairy. Feed your body when it is hungry, but stop when you already feel satisfied.

Aim for variety.

There is nothing wrong with being adventurous about your food. You can pick out different foods from the food groups. Do not stick to one type of food from each group. For example, you do not have to stick to carrots whenever you pick out a vegetable. By choosing a variety of foods to include in your diet, you will be able to take all of the nutrients needed by your body.

You need to pay attention to what you eat because it will help you get the correct balance of the minerals, vitamins, and other nutrients that your body needs. Eating healthy can and will give you more energy, it will also make you feel better. By eating healthy, you can prevent the onset of a lot of health problems, including the following:

High blood pressure or hypertension

Diabetes Mellitus Type 2

Heart Disease

Some cancers

Healthy eating is not a fad. It actually means having to make changes wherein you get to live and enjoy your life better and healthier. Fad diets are those that are temporary in nature. Most of these fad diets make you give up a lot of foods which make you feel hungry and think about eating those foods you had to give up. Once you stop dieting, there is a high tendency that you will overeat and will have to start all over again. By eating healthy and having a balanced diet, your body will be more satisfied. If you add in physical activity to the mix, you will also be able to achieve a healthy weight. You will most likely be able to maintain that healthy weight with a balanced, healthy eating compared to the fad diets.

So, how do you make eating healthy a habit? First of all, list down the different reasons why you want to change. Do you wish for better health? Do you want to feel better about yourself? Do you want to be a role model to your children? Once you have completed your list, think about the little changes that you can incorporate into your daily life. Be sure to choose the ones that you can do long-term.

Remember that you cannot change everything all at once.

Create a long-term goal, like having one vegetarian lunch or dinner in a week.

Come up with an easy goal that you can reach, such as eating a piece of fruit every day.

It also helps to get support from other people. The more support that a person has, the easier and faster it will be to incorporate changes into his or her life. You can ask your friends and family to practice healthy eating together with you. You can even ask them to help prepare meals, share delicious and healthy recipes, as well as cooking tips. If you need help to get started, you can try asking a registered dietitian or your physician. There are also online groups that help promote and support healthy eating. You can read about the success stories of people on the sites, too.

CHAPTER 3

Recipes for Healthy Snacking

Healthy eating starts by substituting healthier alternatives for the usual foods that you eat that contain high amounts of salt, fat, and sugar. Many people commit the mistake of eating healthy meals, but they also revert to eating snacks that are unhealthy, such as chips, sodas, and a lot more. In terms of healthy eating, it is important to make wise decisions, including snack choices. This chapter will help you find different snacks that will help you make healthier choices. Read on to find out more!

Edamame and Cranberry Mix

This recipe makes 1 cup and may be stored up to 5 days in an airtight container. You can place this on your desk for easy reach whenever you feel like snacking.

Ingredients:

- A cup of frozen shelled edamame
- 1 tsp of extra virgin olive oil
- ¼ cup of dried cranberries
- Salt

Steps:

1. Let the shelled edamame thaw.
2. Heat the oven to 425 degrees Fahrenheit.
3. On a baking sheet, place the edamame. Take the oil and

drizzle on top.

4. Add some salt on the edamame.

5. Place the baking sheet into the oven to roast. Be sure to stir occasionally until the edamame turns crisp and golden in color. This takes about 20 to 22 minutes.

6. Let the edamame cool. Toss in the cranberries and mix well. Store in an airtight container.

Frozen Fruit Salad8

This recipe makes use of common fruits. You will be surprised as to how tasty and delicious this simple snack is!

Ingredients:

- 2 cups of seedless green grapes
- 2 cups of seedless red grapes
- 2 bananas

Steps:

1. After peeling the bananas, slice them crosswise, about ½-inch thick.

2. On a small baking sheet (rimmed), place the grapes and bananas in a single layer. Pop into the freezer until they are all frozen.

3. Divide the frozen pieces into 4 bowls and serve.

4. If you are working outside the house, you can place the fruit in a little plastic bag or container. Pop the bag in the freezer at your workplace, then take it out when you are ready to eat your snack.

Homemade Popcorn

To those who wish to snack on grains, popcorn is actually a whole grain snack. It is known to contain low calories and contains the crunchiness that people seek. However, the pre-packed popcorn in the grocery stores is a lot more expensive and contains additives that are not good for the health. This recipe will help you take out the unnecessary add-ons and come up with a snack that will keep you full, at just a fraction of the cost of supermarket popcorn.

Ingredients:

- ¼ cup of popcorn kernels
- 1 teaspoon of olive oil
- 1 brown paper bag

Steps:

1. In a bowl, place the kernels. Add in the oil. Mix well to make sure that all of the kernels are oiled.

2. Transfer the kernels into a brown paper bag. Fold the top part a few times and add some tape.

3. Place the paper bag in the microwave, with the folded side up. Cook the popcorn for 2 to 3 minutes, or when there is a 5-second interval between pops.

4. You may add some sea salt for flavor, but you can also eat this plain.

Banana Quesadillas

This recipe is very tasty and makes a great snack after work. This serves 2.

Ingredients:

- 1 banana (ripe)
- 2 tortillas, whole grain
- 1 tbsp peanut butter or any other type of nut butter
- Some chocolate chips (This is optional.)

Steps:

1. Using a potato masher or a fork, mash the banana in a bowl.
2. Spread the peanut or nut butter on one tortilla, followed by the mashed banana. If you like it with chocolate, add in a few chocolate chips then top with the remaining tortilla.
3. Warm the quesadilla in the microwave for about 20 seconds or so. You can take this to work and warm it in your office microwave or simply eat it right away.

Cinnamon Ora8nges

- ¼ tsp ground cinnamon
- 4 navel oranges
- 1 tbsp sugar
- 2 tbsps lemon juice
- 2 tbsps orange juice

Steps:

1. Using a sharp knife, take out the rind of the oranges, as well as the white pith. Cut the oranges horizontally into about 5 to 6 slices. Arrange the slices onto 4 plates.

2. In a bowl, whisk the cinnamon, lemon and orange juice, and the sugar. Be sure to mix them well.

3. Once done, spoon the syrup on the orange slices.

Muesli Scones

You can pack some of these scones for work. You can bring along some butter and honey to put on top when you are going to eat already.

Ingredients:

- 2 cups of self-rising flour
- 1 tbsp caster sugar
- ½ cup of plain flour
- 30 grams of unsalted butter, chilled then chopped
- ¾ cup of toasted muesli
- ¾ cup of milk (low-fat)
- Some honey and unsalted butter when serving

Steps:

1. Preheat the oven to 250 degrees Celsius. Using cooking spray, grease lightly a 19-cm square cake pan.

2. Sift the flours and the sugar inside a large bowl. Add in the

chopped butter. With your fingertips, rub the butter into the flour until the mixture looks like breadcrumbs.

3. Add in the milk a little at a time. Using a flat-blade knife, stir in the milk to create a soft dough. If needed, you may add more milk.

4. On a lightly-floured surface, turn the dough. Fold in the muesli and knead everything together gently until the dough is formed.

5. Halve the dough. Shape one half into a circle, about 2 centimeters thick. With a 5-centimeter glass or cutter, cut circles from the rounded dough. Repeat the step with the scraps and the remaining dough. Transfer the shaped scones onto the prepared pan.

6. Let the scones bake for about 12 to 15 minutes or until they turn golden. Add butter and honey on top when you are ready to eat.

Classic Hummus

This all-around dip also goes well as a dressing to various salads or a simple dip for vegetables like cucumbers and celery. This also goes well with warm pita or tortillas.

Ingredients:

-   1 15-ounce can of chickpeas, drained and then rinsed
-   2 tablespoons of lemon juice
-   1 garlic clove, chopped
-   ¼ teaspoon of salt

- 2 tablespoons of tahini or sesame paste
- 2 tablespoons of water
- 2 tablespoons of olive oil
- Paprika (This is optional.)

Steps:

1. Combine chickpeas, salt, garlic, tahini, lemon juice, water, and olive oil in a food processor. Let everything pulse until the mixture becomes smooth. Scrape the sides of the processor from time to time.

2. Season the hummus with olive oil, salt, and paprika if needed and desired. You can refrigerate this for up to 7 days.

Vegetable Tortilla Spirals

If you want to incorporate vegetables into your snacks, this is the perfect recipe for you.

Ingredients:

- 2 whole grain tortillas
- 150 grams of hummus
- 1 big carrot, peeled, then grated coarsely
- 1 cup of broccoli and alfalfa sprouts (about 60 grams)

Steps:

1. Spread the hummus onto the tortillas.
2. Sprinkle the broccoli and alfalfa sprouts and carrot on the hummus.

3. Roll up the tortilla to form a log. Do the same with the other tortilla.

4. Cut the rolls into 4 portions. Serve. You can place this in a small container to take to work.

Cherry-Chocolate Snack Bars

Most of the cereal bars that are available commercially are actually packed with a lot of preservatives and other substances that are not good for the body. This recipe will help you come up with your own homemade cereal bar that is crunchy, chewy, and delicious. It is packed with nuts, seeds, fruit, and chocolate! You may use any type of dried fruit for this recipe if you do not want to stick to cherries or cranberries alone. This makes 16 bars.

Ingredients:

- 2 ½ cups of puffed wheat cereal, unsweetened
- 1/3 cup of salted roasted pepitas
- ¼ cup of dried cranberries or cherries, chopped coarsely
- ½ cup of pecan halves, chopped medium-fine
- 1 tablespoon of ground flaxseeds
- 2 tablespoons of sesame seeds
- ½ teaspoon of vanilla extract
- ½ cup of bittersweet chocolate, finely chopped
- ½ cup of honey
- 1/8 teaspoon of salt

Steps:

1. Preheat the oven to 300 degrees Fahrenheit. In the lower third part of the oven, take a rack and place it there.

2. Line a square pan (8-inch) with some parchment paper. Be sure to let it hang on the opposite sides.

3. In a large bowl, mix the sesame seeds, pecans, cereal, cranberries or cherries, pepitas, and the ground flaxseeds. Mix well.

4. In a small saucepan, combine the salt, honey, and vanilla. Warm everything on medium heat while stirring. Stop when the honey becomes a lot more fluid and the salt has already dissolved. Pour the mixture onto the dry ingredients. Fold the mixture until the dry ingredients have been coated by honey. Leave the mixture to cool for 5 minutes or so.

5. Fold in the chocolate until everything is evenly distributed. Scrape the cereal mixture and transfer it into the prepared pan. Using a fork, spread the mixture evenly, using the back of the fork to press down on the mixture. You may also use parchment paper on top of the mixture and press firmly down.

6. Place the pan in the oven and bake for about 35 minutes, or until the top turns golden brown. Run the sides of the pan with the knife to detach the bars from the sides. Let it cool on a wire rack at room temperature for about an hour. Lift the ends of the parchment paper to take out the bars.

7. Gently take out the parchment. With a heavy knife, divide the "cake" into 16 squares or bars. Take a piece or more to work as a handy and tasty snack.

Sugar Snap Peas
with Kale Dip

If you want to shy away for a while from typical salads and blended greens, this is another way of eating your vegetables!

Ingredients:

- 2 cups of trimmed sugar snap peas
- 3 cups of kale leaves, thinly sliced
- 1 tablespoon of extra-virgin olive oil
- 1 cup of cottage cheese, low-fat
- 1 clove of garlic, thinly sliced
- 1 tablespoon of fresh lemon juice
- A pinch of red pepper flakes
- Salt (coarse)

Steps:

1. Over medium heat, heat the oil inside a pan. Add in the kale and garlic. Season these with salt. Cook everything with the cover on. Stir the kale from time to time until everything becomes tender. This takes about 3 to 4 minutes. Let the leaves cool.

2. Transfer the leaves into a food processor. Add in the cottage cheese and let them puree until very smooth. Season with lemon juice and pepper flakes.

3. In a big pot, boil some water (well-salted) to a boil. Add in the peas and let them cook until they turn green and tender. This takes about 1 to 2 minutes. Transfer the peas to an ice-

bath right away. Drain well.

4. Take some of the peas and dip and place in a container for work.

Apricot-Date-Banana Oat Bars

This is a snack that both children and adults will like.

Ingredients:

- 3 cups of rolled oats (traditional-style)
- 3 bananas, large and ripe
- ¼ cup of dried apricots, finely chopped
- ¼ cup of dried dates, finely chopped
- 1 tsp of ground cinnamon
- ¼ cup of slivered almonds
- 1 ½ tsps of vanilla extract

Steps:

1. Preheat the oven to 180 degrees Celsius. Grease a slice pan (16 centimeters x 25.5 centimeters). Line it with parchment or baking paper, with an extra 2 centimeters that extends above the edges.

2. Using a fork or potato masher, mash the bananas until everything is smooth.

3. Fold in the vanilla, dates, apricots, oats, cinnamon, and almonds. Stir everything until well-combined. Spoon the mixture onto the prepared pan. With the spoon, press the mixture firmly and evenly onto the pan.

4. Bake the mixture until it turns golden, or for about 30 to 35 minutes. Let the mixture cool completely. Cut this into small bars or squares. Store in an airtight container.

Flaxseed and Onion Crackers

These crackers go well with any type of cheese, such as Brie. These also go well with hummus topped with some vegetables.

Ingredients:

- 1 ½ cups of all-purpose flour, with extra for dusting
- ¼ cup of whole golden flaxseed
- ¼ cup of ground golden flaxseed
- 1 tbsp plus 1 tsp of onion, grated finely
- ½ tsp of coarse salt, with extra for seasoning if needed
- ½ tsp of baking powder
- 1 tbsp plus 1 tsp of fresh flat-leaf parsley, finely chopped
- 1 egg white, large, beaten lightly
- 2 tbsps of unsalted butter, softened
- ½ cup of of skim milk
- Pepper, freshly ground

Steps:

1. Preheat the oven to 325 degrees Fahrenheit. The racks should be found in the lower and upper thirds of the oven.

2. In a bowl of an electric mixer (use the paddle attachment), mix the ground and whole flaxseed, salt, baking powder,

flour, and butter. Mix everything on medium speed, until the mixture looks like breadcrumbs. This takes about 2 minutes. Mix in the parsley and onion. On low speed, add in the milk. Mix until everything comes together.

3. Divide the dough into 2 halves. Roll each piece on a surface that has been lightly floured. Roll them out into 9-inch squares, of about 1/8 inch thick. Transfer these to two baking sheets. Cut the squares with a pastry knife or fluted pastry wheel into about 30 mini squares. This would be about 1 ½ inch-squares.

4. Brush the top with the egg white, then season with pepper and more salt if you wish. Place the baking sheets in the oven and bake for about 20 minutes, or when they are already slightly firm. Switch the positions of the sheets and flip the crackers. Bake the crackers for 18 to 20 minutes more.

5. Take the crackers out to cool on wire racks. Serve with your favorite dip, such as hummus or kale dip. You can also snack on these plain.

Parsnip-Carrot-Zucchini Frittata Fingers

Ingredients:

- ½ cup of grated green zucchini, firmly packed
- ½ cup of grated parsnip, firmly packed
- ½ cup of grated carrot, firmly packed

- 2 teaspoons of light olive oil
- Some melted butter to grease the pan
- 3 eggs, whisked lightly
- 2 green shallots (ends trimmed), chopped finely
- 1/3 cup of tasty cheese, coarsely grated
- 1 tablespoon of flour, sifted
- 2 tablespoons of fresh parsely, finely chopped

Steps:

1. Preheat the oven to 180 degrees Celsius. Using the melted butter, brush a square and shallow 18.5 centimeter base cake pan. Line the bottom and the 2 opposite sides using baking paper (non-stick) with about 2 centimeters extra hanging from the sides.

2. In a medium saucepan, heat the oil over medium heat. Add in the shallots, zucchini, parsnip, and carrot. Let everything cook for 4 to 5 minutes, until the vegetables become soft. Stir everything to avoid burning the vegetables. Take them out of the heat and leave to cool.

3. In a large bowl, mix the flour, egg, vegetable mixture, parsley, and cheese. Stir everything until well-combined.

4. Spoon everything into the prepared pan and smoothen the surface. Let the mixture bake in the oven for about 12 minutes or until everything is set. Take out from the oven and leave to cool for about 10 minutes.

5. Taking the paper that extended from the edges, lift the frittata. Put on a plate and leave to cool completely.

6. Cut the frittata into 12 fingers.

CHAPTER 4

More Tips on How to Eat and Snack Healthy: Important Things to Remember

A balanced and healthy diet is important for maintaining good health. It will also help you feel better about yourself. Eating healthy does not need to be difficult, just remember the following:

Eat the right amount of calories according to your lifestyle. This will help you find the correct balance between the energy that you use and the energy you ingest. If you drink or eat too much, you will gain weight. If you drink or eat too little, you will then lose weight. On average, men need about 2,500 calories every day, while women need about 2,000 calories a day. Many adults commit the mistake of eating more than what they need.

It is important to eat a wide variety of foods. This will help ensure that you are getting a balanced diet. Your body will be able to get all of the needed nutrients this way.

Here are practical tips that can help you remember what to eat when eating healthy. These can also help you come up with better and healthier decisions:

Base what you eat on good starches.

Starchy foods are the primary source of energy for the body. Include the wholegrain varieties in your diet over potatoes and other refined carbohydrates. Whole grains help you feel more satisfied longer as they contain more fiber.

Eat more fruits and vegetables.

It is said that the average person should consume at least 5 portions of different vegetables and fruit daily. Learn how to incorporate fruits and vegetables into your diet to be healthier.

Consume more fish.

Fish gives the body protein and it also has many minerals and vitamins. You can start with a goal of eating at least 2 servings per week, with one serving from oily fish. Oily fish like salmon, herring, fresh tuna, and sardines contain omega-3 fats, which are good for your health.

Stay away from refined sugars and saturated fat.

Though you need fat in your diet, you have to pay attention as to the type and amount of fat that you are ingesting. Cut down on the foods that contains saturated fats, such as lard and butter. Stay away from sugary foods and drinks, too, including alcohol.

Take less salt.

If buying food, check the food labels for the sodium content. More than 1.5 grams of salt in every 100 grams translates to the fact that it contains a lot of salt. Children over 11 years and adults should not consume more than 6 grams of sodium every day.

Do not skip breakfast.

Many people think that skipping breakfast will help them achieve a healthier weight. However, studies have shown that eating breakfast can actually help dieters control their weight. It is important to include a healthy breakfast in a balanced diet.

Live an active lifestyle to get a healthy weight.

A healthy diet will help you achieve a healthy weight, especially when paired with exercise. Physical activity can help speed up weight loss or can help a person bulk up. Exercise does not necessarily mean that you should spend hours in the gym, but you can also find other activities that you can easily fit into your schedule.

Get hydrated.

Remember that you need to drink approximate 1.2 liters of water daily in order to prevent dehydration. Avoid drinking alcoholic and sugary drinks. When the temperature spikes up or when you have an active lifestyle, you will need more than 1.2 liters. Stick to water, milk, and fresh fruit juices.

Conclusion

Thank you again for purchasing this book!

I hope this book was able to help you to discover a healthier lifestyle through eating highly nutritious and very tasty snacks.

The next step is to try out some of the recipes in this book, so you can find out that healthy eating does not mean you have to eat boring and bland foods every day. With the tips and recipes in this book, you will find that eating healthy can actually be fun and exciting.

Finally, if you enjoyed this book, please take the time to share your thoughts and post a review on Amazon. It'd be greatly appreciated!

Thank you and good luck!

Dr. Daniel Amos

http://www.AfflatusPublishing.com

Check Out Afflatus Publishing On Facebook

HEALTHY SNACKS FOR HEALTHY KIDS

SUPER QUICK, SURE-TO-PLEASE HEALTHY SNACKS ON A SHOESTRING BUDGET

Introduction

I want to thank you and congratulate you for purchasing the book, "Healthy Snacks for Healthy Kids."

This book contains proven steps and strategies on how to provide your kids and your family with the healthiest meals possible so you can all live a healthy and happy life.

This book is fantastic as a guide to keeping your kids healthy, including breakfast recipes, lunch foods, after-school snacks, and dinner ideas that your kids and your family will enjoy!

Thanks again for purchasing this book, and I hope you enjoy it!

The Importance of Raising Healthy Kids

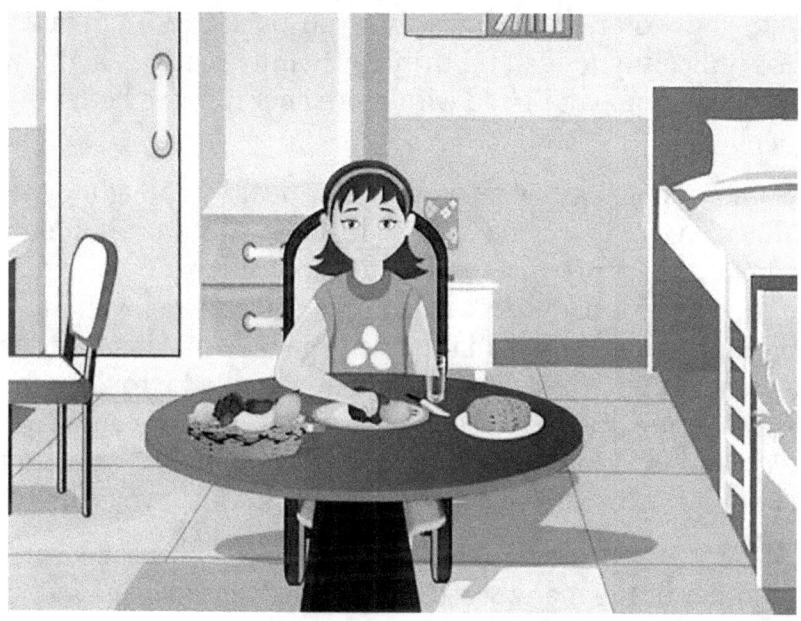

As parents, it is our job to ensure that the food consumed by our children is as healthy as possible. The saying "You are what you eat" is very true, and the importance of a healthy diet must be instilled into kids at a young age; otherwise, they could be doomed to a life of unhealthy living. It isn't always easy to get kids to eat things that we see as being good for them, but there are a few tricks you can use to make eating healthy seem fun.

The path to living a healthy lifestyle with healthy children begins in the womb. Of course, you want to eat healthy when you are carrying your child and you want everything to be perfect and your child to come into this world healthy. That sense of keeping your child healthy should not stop once they are born; to have a healthy and happy child, you must live as a healthy family. If you are accustomed to processed foods, sugary treats, and sodas, it is past the time to give these things up. After a while, you won't even notice that you once had a craving for these unhealthy foods and drinks. Healthy, natural living will provide you and your child with more energy and a better overall feeling.

So how do you know if something is healthy enough for your family or not? Always read the labels and check for hidden ingredients. Many products will say in large letters, on the front of the container or bag, 100% natural; however, when you flip the container around and read the fine print, you may find artificial sweeteners and other things that can actually be toxic to your body. Organic is always best, but in some cases, it can be quite pricey, so shop around and find a favorite shop or favorite brand that you can trust for all of your edible products you purchase for your household.

Another of the many reasons that you want to keep you kids on a healthy, natural diet is the risk of allergens that are associated with some foods. Some of the preservatives and GMOs placed in our foods sold in grocery stores are big contributors to the onset of asthma and other allergy-related problems that so many children nowadays suffer from. It makes sense that these health problems are a result of our food and our environment, as throughout history, there are very few recordings of these problems in children or adults for that matter.

A lot of major health issues could be cleared up, if only more people lived a life full of whole and organic foods only. Nothing that is processed should ever be allowed in your pantry. Just imagine the process that these products, such as Twinkies and HoHos, go through before they reach your kitchen. The thought can be sickening. These are most definitely NOT naturally occurring substances and therefore our bodies are not made to digest and properly break them down. These types of foods, if you can call them foods, are really not suitable for human consumption and definitely not for a small child.

If you raise your child or children to be more health conscious than most average Americans, you stand a much better chance of them continuing this behavior throughout their entire lives. This is the ultimate goal when you are raising your child, to ensure that they are, and will continue to be, healthy and happy throughout their lifetime. Health and happiness begin with clean living. This means also no smoking, drinking, or taking of any other toxic substances that some people choose to put into their bodies.

Always remember that your body is your temple. Yes, it sounds a bit cliché; however, you can't change the fact, and the fact is that your body gets what you put into it. Therefore, in order to raise your child into a healthy and happy adult, you must start teaching them while they are young the best way to maintain being healthy by monitoring what they consume.

Fun Snacks That Kids Will Love

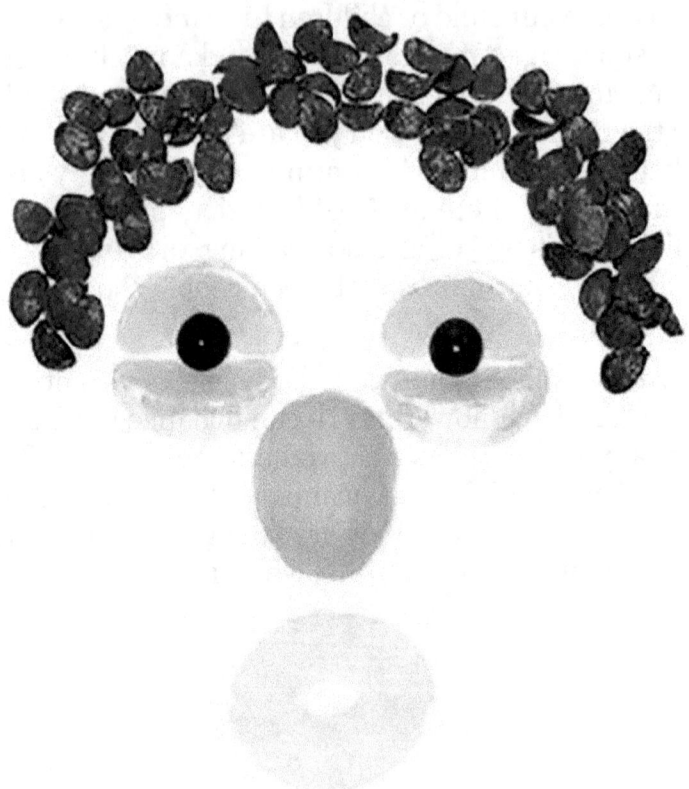

So now that you have established a better understanding of why it is so very important to keep your children eating naturally grown and nonprocessed foods, the question you are probably asking yourself is how to get them to like it. There are tons of fun snack ideas that kids will be very fond of and grow to love.

Here are examples of some of the top healthy snacks for kids. These are things that you can send with your child to school, as a snack, or have when they get home. All of the following foods are naturally occurring in our environment and therefore easily digestible, making both you and your child happier. Nobody likes to have an upset tummy, especially children.

Fun After-School Snacks

1.) Apples Cut Up with a Peanut Butter Spread

Everyone loves apples, well almost everyone. If you child likes apples, this will be a perfect snack to have when they get home and are starting on homework. You can either spread the peanut butter over the cut up apple pieces or leave the peanut butter as a dip. Either way, your child will benefit from the natural goodness of the fruit and the protein in the peanut butter. This type of snack food will give your child better and more sustained energy to go out and play, or whatever they enjoy doing after school, than some processed, sugary snack would. To make this even more enjoyable for your child, let them help. Kids learn by example, so always try to set a good example when it comes to your health. Allow your child to pick out the apple and "help" as you cut it up. Then, you can give them a choice either peanut butter spread or dip; this will give your child not only the benefit of having a healthy snack but also the satisfaction of helping out in the kitchen.

2.) **Ants on a Log: Also Known as Peanut Butter and Celery Topped with Raisins**

This snack is extremely easy for anyone to make, and yes, it has peanut butter as well. Peanut butter is an excellent source of protein, and unless there is an allergy issue, almost all kids love peanut butter. This is a great way to get your kids to try celery, which without the peanut butter and the fun name, "ants on a log," kids may be more hesitant to even consider trying celery. I know my boys wouldn't have any part of celery until I made them this fun snack. Again, it is important to let your child help you in the process of making after-school snacks, it gives them the feeling that they did something themselves, and it is a great bonding activity you can share with your child.

3.) **After-School Smoothie as an Alternative to Ice Cream**

Back in the old days, you may have had parents or grandparents who would take you to get ice cream as an after-school treat, but in today's world, that just won't work. Ice cream is full of processed sugars and overall is just not a healthy sack for kids. This natural and healthy smoothie recipe will keep your kids' sweet tooth satisfied and give you the comfort of knowing that you have provided your child with a healthy snack that they will enjoy.

Simply take low-fat milk, frozen strawberries, and a banana, place the ingredients into a blender, and blend until smooth and creamy.

Your child will love helping in making this fun snack and you will enjoy it too. These smoothies are best on a hot day, either after school or when your child takes a break from playing outside. The fresh fruits will give your child nutrients he or she needs, and the calcium in the milk will help in building strong bones.

4.) **Fruity Cheese Kabobs**

A new twist on an old concept that your kids will love creating with you. Pick out a few of your child's favorite fruits (berries work best for this fun treat) and select some low-fat cheese, the kind that comes in blocks that can be cut into fun shapes. Get a few kabob sticks, long or short, it doesn't really matter, whichever you think is best suited for your child's age and appetite. I suggest avoiding metal kabob sticks, as these could prove to be dangerous to your child.

Select your chosen fruits and berries and set aside. Take your blocks of cheese and any fun-shaped, but small in size, cookie cutters and cut out 5–10 pieces of cheese with your desired cookie cutter and let your child lay their design out on a paper plate or cutting board. This is also a great way to let your child express themselves artistically while creating a fun after-school snack and promoting quality time together.

Slide the cheeses and fruits onto the kabob sticks in whatever order your child has laid out (you should probably do this part, to avoid any boo-boos).

Now, your child has their very own version of shish kabobs, only much healthier and more fun to make and likely more appetizing to a child than steak and potatoes. You can mix this up any way you like, or you can make strictly fruit kabobs, mixing different colors and varieties of fruits and berries or strictly cheese kabobs made from different shapes. This is one afternoon snack your child is sure to look forward to when they get home for the day. The added benefits of fruits and berries are the antioxidant properties in the fruit, and the cheese will give your child a daily dose of calcium, to promote strong bones. This one is an all-time favorite in our household.

Healthy Breakfasts to Start Your Kids' Day Off Right

Everyone knows that the key to a great day is a great breakfast. Start your child's day off right with a healthy breakfast that will sustain their hunger until lunchtime and give them the energy they need to do well in class. Here are a few healthy breakfast recipes that are easy to make and you can have your child make these with you also. A great idea is to make breakfast the night before, that way you have it already prepared, just in case you are running late, which is something that is inevitable when you have kids.

1.) **Blueberry and Maple Syrup Muffins**

Ingredients

- 1 cup whole wheat flour
- 1/2 cup maple syrup
- 1/3 cup flaxseed
- 1 cup nonfat buttermilk
- 3/4 cup all-purpose flour
- 1/4 cup canola oil
- 1/3 tsp. baking soda
- 2 tsp. fresh orange zest
- 1/4 tsp. salt
- 1 tbsp. orange juice
- 2 large eggs

- 1 1/2 cups fresh blueberries
- 1 tbsp. sugar
- 1 tsp. nutmeg

Steps

1. Preheat oven to 400 degrees and coat your muffin pan with nonstick cooking spray.

2. Grind flaxseed in a clean coffee grinder or blender; add all ingredients, other than the blueberries, into large mixing bowl; and blend until well mixed.

3. Next, fold the fresh blueberries into the mix and scoop the batter into your muffin pan.

4. Let cook for 15–25 minutes and allow to cool for at least 5 minutes.

5. Place the muffins in sandwich bags and have them ready for the following morning. This is one breakfast that your child will really love and will get the benefits of fresh fruit and flax seed, which is full of omega-3 fatty acids, an essential part of a healthy diet. Your child will think they are getting a treat and you will know that it really is healthy.

2.) **English Muffin Egg Pizza Bites**

This breakfast will give your child the perfect balance of carbs and proteins to get them on their way, full and happy. Eggs are an excellent source of protein, while the English muffins provide great carbs. The best part about this breakfast is your child will think they are getting a pizza like treat first thing in the morning; this makes everyone happy.

Ingredients

- 4 small English muffins
- Grated mozzarella
- Olive oil
- A dash of oregano for each muffin
- 1 tomato cut into slices
- 1 tsp. kosher salt
- 2 hard-boiled eggs

Steps

1. Cook eggs until they are hard boiled.
2. Toast your English muffins and place on baking rack in halves.
3. Drizzle olive oil, layer the tomato slices, place 1/2 hard-boiled egg on each muffin, sprinkle some grated mozzarella, and top it off with the oregano and kosher salt.
4. Broil for 5 minutes or until the cheese melts and the muffins begin to brown.
5. Allow muffins to cool for about 5 minutes and serve. This recipe is guaranteed to send your kids off to school happy.

3.) **Oatmeal with Fresh Blueberries and Orange Juice**

This recipe is simple, quick, and easy. Whole grain oatmeal is one of nature's healthiest foods and kids love it. Make a bowl of your child's desired size and add in some fresh blueberries, raspberries, strawberries, or whatever kind of berries you have in the fridge that your child likes. Stir the fruit and oatmeal all together and serve with a nice big glass of orange juice. You couldn't ask for anything easier or more filling for your child's breakfast, and it is a really convenient way for you to start their day off right.

4.) **Whole Grain Waffles with Peanut Butter**

Yes, we are back to the peanut butter again. Peanut butter makes a great substitute for syrup, especially when you are in a rush. Although there are many choices when it comes to waffles, steer clear from the flavored and sugary ones, these are not the healthiest and contain processed sugars that will cause your child to crash midmorning, which could lead to poor behavior in class.

Toast your whole grain waffles and spread peanut butter on top. Some kids like to make a sandwich out of it, which can be a fun way to get your child to eat their breakfast before getting into your car with the sticky peanut butter and all. The whole grains are excellent for your child, and the peanut butter will provide protein to get him or her off to a great start and full of energy for the day.

5.) **Cowboy Eggs**

This is a simple breakfast that your kids are sure to love. All you need are 2 pieces of whole wheat bread and 2 eggs. Using a small cup or cookie cutter, cut out the inner circle of the 2 pieces of bread, butter the edges (light/nonfat butter), and crack the egg right in the middle of the circle. Cook on stovetop on medium-low setting until the egg has cooked enough to flip over. Cook opposite side for approx. 1 minute and viola! Cowboy eggs. Your child will get a healthy dose of protein from the eggs and carbs from the bread; you can even make mini sandwiches for their lunch box or a snack out of the inner circles of the bread. Perfectly simple hot breakfast to get your little one off to a great start and keep him or her full until lunchtime or snack time at school. This is my youngest son's very favorite breakfast choice.

Healthy Lunch Ideas for Kids

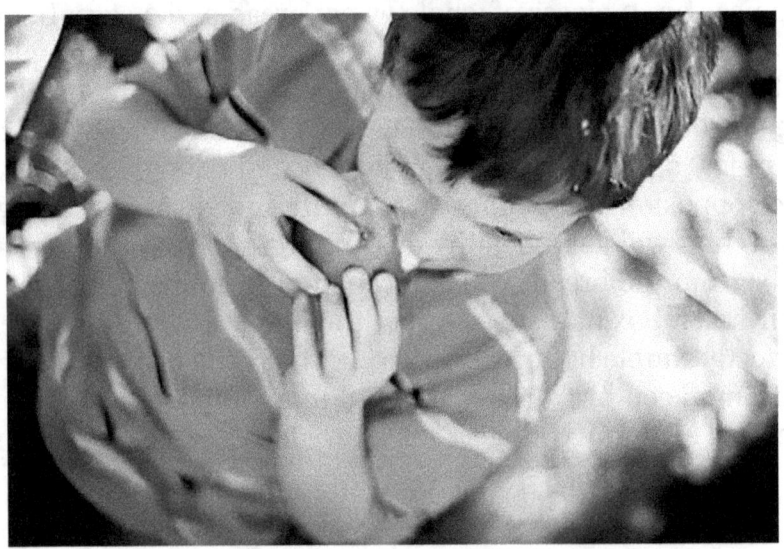

Lunchtime can be a difficult time to ensure that your child has a healthy meal, with the uncertainty of what goes into their school lunches and the possibility of kids trading foods; you never know what they may end up eating. Luckily, you can pack your child's lunch with things that are not only healthy but tasty as well. If you figure out what healthy foods your child likes the most, they will be less likely to trade off with a friend for something that you may or may not approve of. Here is a list of healthy foods to place into your child's lunch pail to ensure he or she has a great lunch.

Grapes – What kid doesn't love grapes? Pack a baggie full in their lunch and rest assured that your child will be getting their fill of nutrient-rich fruits in their lunch.

Oranges – Oranges are a great addition to your kids' lunch box; they are packed full of vitamin C, which supports a healthy immune system. This is really important for school kids who are exposed to the germs and viruses of all the other kids around them on a daily basis. Plus, as an added bonus, kids love to make funny faces with the orange peels, when cut into slices, which will pretty much guarantee that your child will be eating their orange.

Healthy granola bars – These come in whole grains but are disguised as candy bars, sneaky, but a great way to give your child's lunch a healthy boost. Some even come with chocolate drizzle on top, which definitely ensures they won't be trading it out for another snack.

Teddy Grahams (whole wheat) – This is another sneaky ploy to integrate some naturally healthy food into your child's diet. They will love the Teddy Grahams and you will love the nutritional value.

Bananas – Simple and easy to throw in a lunch box and no packaging needed. The potassium in bananas will keep your child's growing pains at bay while keeping them healthy by adding more fruit to their diet.

Whole grain bread – Never buy white bread; for my kids, it is always wheat for all of their sandwiches. The more whole grains you can get your child to eat, the better. If your child is resistant to "brown bread," as my son was at first, try the white wheat version; you get all the same nutrients without the processed flour and it comes in white.

Peanut butter – Yes again, peanut butter is a staple in a kid's diet and a great way to provide protein for their growing muscles and bodies.

Pizza with a whole grain crust – What kid doesn't love to pull a slice of pizza out of their lunch box when all of their friends have the same old sandwiches? This is a treat, as well as a great ploy to add some extra nutrition to their diet!

Organic applesauce – You can get all sorts of different flavors of organic applesauce that comes in convenient little containers that won't spill if dropped. My kids love these and so do their friends; I am not a fan, but kids seem to love them.

Juice – Don't send your child to school with money for a soda, ever. Send natural juices that are inexpensive and come in packs of 12–18. I like to send 2 with my kids, just in case they get thirsty later in the day. This ensures that they will not be venturing off to the soda machine.

Once you have determined what your child's favorite healthy alternatives to sugary sweets are, you can mix it up and provide them with the best and most healthy lunch possible, making sure that even if you aren't around, they still eat nutritious foods.

Healthy Dinners for the Whole Family

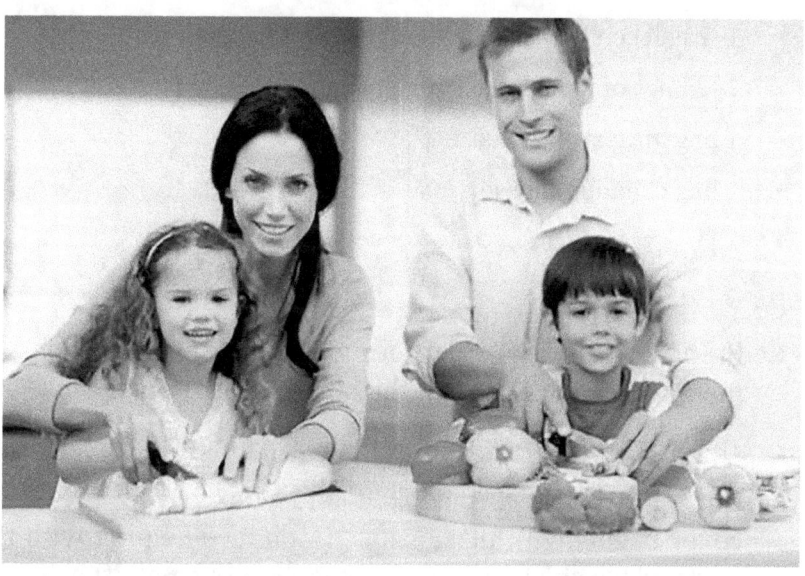

If your child is picky when it comes to dinner, have no fear; there are plenty of kid-friendly family recipes that will satisfy mom and dad, as well as the kiddos. The best part is that most of these recipes are easy to make and won't require much cleanup. I think it is a good practice to get your kids involved and offer them one night per week that they can choose their dinner or the family dinner. I fell into the trap of cooking separate meals for everyone because of having a house full of picky eaters, but with these yummy dishes, you are sure to find something that works for everyone.

1.) Chicken and Cheese Bagel Pizza

Ingredients

- 1–2 chicken breasts (depending on your family size)
- 1–2 bags of plain bagels (again, depending on your family size)
- 1 bag mozzarella cheese
- 1 bag cheddar cheese
- 1 jar pizza sauce

Steps

1. Preheat oven to 405 degrees and place chicken in glass or metal pan and cook until the middle is no longer pink.

2. Toast your desired amount of bagels in toaster.

3. Once the chicken is cooked and your bagels are ready, cover bagels with pizza sauce (kids love helping with this part); place chicken on top of bagels, along with the desired amount of cheese; and broil until the cheese is melty and the entire pizza bagel is slightly crispy.

4. This is a quick and easy meal that your whole family will enjoy. You can even make a chicken–pizza bagel sandwich out of your creation. Once a week, let your kids have fun with their food; now, I don't mean food fights or any of that nonsense, but if your child wants to make it a pizza sandwich, let them. Being able to express their creativity is one of the most important parts of growing up, even when it comes to chicken–pizza bagel sandwiches.

2.) Whole Wheat Taco Pizzas

Yes, another pizza recipe, kids love pizza, and I have found various different ways to offer it to them without all the grease that you get in delivery style pizzas.

Ingredients

- 1 package whole wheat tortilla wraps
- 1–2 bags mozzarella cheese
- 1 jar pizza sauce
- 1 package lean pepperoni

Steps

1. There really isn't much to the preparation of this dish – simply fill a small bowl with pizza sauce and another with cheese, give your child a spoon and a plate with their tortilla wrap laid out on it, and allow them to spread the sauce all over the tortilla. You guessed it! Next comes the cheese. You can place these in the microwave for about 30 seconds to avoid the edges becoming crispy, or if you like it crispy, simply broil for about 5 minutes on high. This really is more of a kid's meal, but you can add any vegetables you like and turn it into a wrap, making everyone happy.

3.) Baked Chicken Nuggets

Every kid loves chicken nuggets, but the drive-through nuggets you get at fast-food restaurants are terrible when it comes to healthy foods. Here is a fantastic recipe that you and your kids will love.

Ingredients

- 16 oz. skinless, boneless chicken breasts (cut into pieces)
- Salt and pepper (according to your tastes)
- 2 tsp. extra virgin olive oil
- 6 tbsp. whole wheat Italian seasoned bread crumbs
- 2 tbsp. parmesan cheese
- Olive oil spray

Steps

1. Preheat oven to 425 degrees and spray your baking sheet with olive oil spray.
2. Place all of your ingredients, except the salt and pepper, into a Ziploc bag that can withstand you shaking it.
3. Add chicken to the bag and shake to mix the breadcrumbs, olive oil, and spices.
4. Remove chicken from the bag and place onto baking sheet.
5. Bake for about 8 minutes on one side and 6–7 minutes on the next side.
6. Allow nuggets to cool for 10–15 minutes and add desired veggies to your families' plates, and you have yourself a healthy dinner that pleases the whole family.

7. Don't be afraid to play around with any of the recipes in this book and mix them up a bit, according to your preferred tastes. It's all about being happy, healthy, and eating together as a family.

4.) Sloppy Joes with Turkey

Everybody loves sloppy joes! They're fun, they're messy, and it is acceptable to eat using your fingers – what more could a kid ask for? This version of the old sloppy joe mix is a bit more health conscious, and it's something the whole family can agree on. Also, another great opportunity to let your little one help out in the kitchen.

Ingredients (for a family of 4, you may adjust accordingly to fit your family size)

- 4 whole wheat hamburger buns
- 2 1/2 tbsp. brown sugar
- 1 lb. ground turkey meat
- 3–4 grated carrots
- 1 can crushed tomatoes
- 3 tbsp. tomato paste
- 1 tsp. Worcestershire sauce
- 1 minced red onion
- 1 tbsp. olive oil
- Salt and Pepper to taste

Steps

1. In large saucepan, on medium, heat olive oil and add carrots and minced onion. Stir occasionally over the course of about 5 minutes, until the onions begin to brown a bit.

2. Add in your tomato paste and stir, allowing to cook for about 5 minutes.

3. Add turkey meat and cook until no pink meat is visible, normally around 5–7 minutes.

4. Add in tomatoes, brown sugar, and Worcestershire sauce and cook all together for approximately 15 minutes. Stir occasionally until your sauce has thickened to the correct consistency for the world's best and healthiest sloppy joes.

5. Allow to cool for about 5–7 minutes and serve on whole wheat hamburger buns with your choice of side vegetables. Broccoli is great because kids like to think of them as little trees, I always get a kick out of my son pretending to be a giant when he eats broccoli. There you have it, in less than 30 minutes (minus cooling period and the time it takes to round up your family for dinnertime) a perfectly healthy, family-friendly meal that everyone is sure to love.

5.) Baked Guacamole Casserole

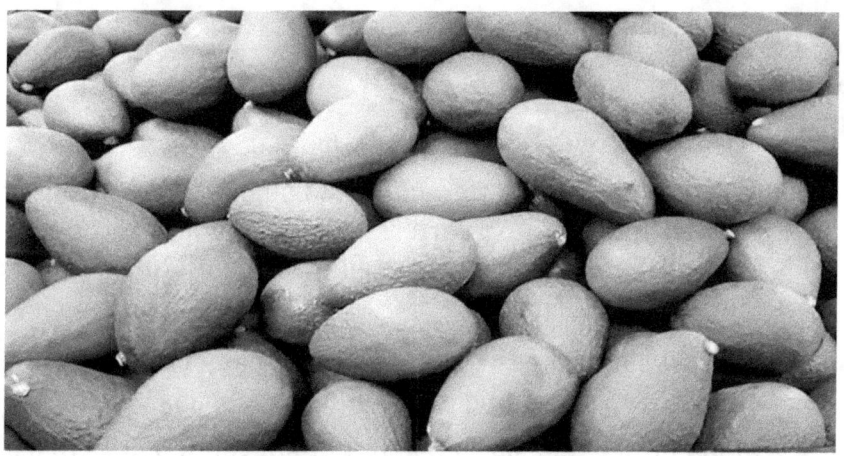

I know what you are thinking – guacamole isn't a meal, it's a side. Am I right? Well, this is my very favorite recipe that I have ever created, and my family agrees, so it must be the best one I've come up with. Even if you don't like guacamole, you will like this. I know this because I greatly dislike guacamole (don't ask why I created this recipe, because I have no clue). Either way, it's good and healthy and makes a great addition to tacos also.

Ingredients

- 3–4 ripe avocados (the darker, the better)
- 1 can black beans
- 1 small container sour cream
- 2 16 oz. bags of Mexican blend cheese
- 1 pouch taco seasoning

- 1/2 red onion
- 1 large jar of salsa
- 1 lb. lean ground beef (optional)

Steps

1. Preheat oven to 405 degrees.

2. In a blender or preferably a Cuisinart, place avocados (peeled and cut into quarters). ***Tip: If your avocados are hard to remove from their peeling, place in the microwave for 30–60 seconds.***

3. Add in 1 bag of cheese, 1/2 container of sour cream, chopped onions, taco seasoning, salsa, and black beans.

4. Blend until you have a creamy, but not soupy, consistency.

5. Pour into glass or metal pan, any size will do, and bake for 10–15 minutes.

6. After you have baked the guacamole, remove from oven and top with cheese.

7. Broil on high for 3–4 minutes or until the cheese has browned slightly but is still melty and delicious looking.

8. Remove from oven and allow to cool for 5–7 minutes, and there you have yourself authentic baked guacamole casserole. A friend, who is also a chef, told me it is odd to bake guacamole in America, but that in Argentina, baked guacamole is an authentic, age old dish. Serve in portions with some chips or roll up in a whole wheat tortilla for a yummy dinner that your family will beg you to make every day for a month.

Conclusion

Thank you again for downloading this book!

I hope this book was able to help you to discover new and inventive ways to keep your family healthy and happy.

The next step is to check your grocery list, as well as your pantry, and fill your cabinets with whole grain foods, fruits, and veggies that will be pleasing to your families' taste buds.

Finally, if you enjoyed this book, please take the time to share your thoughts and post a review on Amazon. It'd be greatly appreciated!

Thank you and good luck!

Victoria Love, Daniel Amos
&
Sylvie Johnstone